COMMOD BODS

COMMOD BODS

EMBODIED HERITAGE, FOODWAYS, AND INDIGENEITY

KASEY JERNIGAN

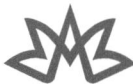

THE UNIVERSITY OF
ARIZONA PRESS

TUCSON

The University of Arizona Press
www.uapress.arizona.edu

We respectfully acknowledge the University of Arizona is on the land and territories of Indigenous peoples. Today, Arizona is home to twenty-two federally recognized tribes, with Tucson being home to the O'odham and the Yaqui. The University strives to build sustainable relationships with sovereign Native Nations and Indigenous communities through education offerings, partnerships, and community service.

ISBN-13: 978-0-8165-5622-9 (hardcover)
ISBN-13: 978-0-8165-5621-2 (paperback)
ISBN-13: 978-0-8165-5623-6 (ebook)

Cover design by Leigh McDonald
Cover art: *Commodities (Food of My People)* © 2025 Zig Jackson / Artists Rights Society (ARS), New York
Typeset by Sara Thaxton in 105/14 Warnock Pro with Helvetica Neue LT Std

Publication of this book is made possible in part through research startup support from The College and Graduate School of Arts & Sciences at the University of Virginia.

Library of Congress Cataloging-in-Publication Data
Names: Jernigan, Kasey, 1978– author
Title: Commod bods : embodied heritage, foodways, and indigeneity / Kasey Jernigan.
Description: [Tucson] : The University of Arizona Press, 2026. | Includes bibliographical references and index.
Identifiers: LCCN 2025013850 (print) | LCCN 2025013851 (ebook) | ISBN 9780816556229 hardcover | ISBN 9780816556212 paperback | ISBN 9780816556236 ebook
Subjects: LCSH: Choctaw Indians—Health and hygiene—Oklahoma | Choctaw Indians—Food—Social aspects—Oklahoma | Food consumption—Social aspects—Oklahoma | Food relief—Social aspects—Oklahoma
Classification: LCC E99.C8 J445 2026 (print) | LCC E99.C8 (ebook)
LC record available at https://lccn.loc.gov/2025013850
LC ebook record available at https://lccn.loc.gov/2025013851

Printed in the United States of America
♾ This paper meets the requirements of ANSI/NISO Z39.48-1992 (Permanence of Paper).

CONTENTS

ILLUSTRATIONS

FIGURES

TABLES

ACKNOWLEDGMENTS

This book carries more than text. It holds memory, kinship, story, gratitude, exhaustion, and care. It was crafted in borrowed hours, in the margins of parenting, grieving, loving, teaching, fighting, and beginning again. Everything in this book exists because I was never alone in the making.

I'm grateful to the University of Arizona Press for taking this project in and walking it toward the world. Deep thanks to Allyson Carter for seeing the shape of this book and championing it with such care and enthusiasm. Thank you, Alana Enriquez, Amanda Krause, Leigh McDonald, and Mikaela Ball for your work behind the scenes to help pull the many pieces of this manuscript together with gentle precision and thoughtfulness. I also want to thank Abby Mogollón, Mary Reynolds, and Cameron Louie for your careful stewardship of the work beyond the pages of the manuscript. Thank you all for making this book feel like itself, even on the outside. To the anonymous reviewers who read this manuscript with care and clarity, thank you. Your feedback was not only thoughtful and incisive, but your readings gave me the courage to bring it fully into the world. Thank you to Zig Jackson (Buffalo Rising) for allowing this layered and powerful image to become the face of the book. Your photograph captures the sentiment of commodity foods with quiet force, making visual so much of what this book aims to articulate.

To my earliest mentors, Tom Leatherman, Jane Anderson, and Lisa Wexler, thank you for being there from the beginning. You guided me to ask the right questions, handed me books that helped me think deeply, and gave me the freedom to explore my ideas while gently shepherding me through the strange architectures of academic research. You taught me not just how to be an academic, but how to be the kind of academic I want to be: one rooted in both rigor and relationality, in freedom and structure, and always accountable to the communities I come from and work alongside.

I'm also deeply grateful to my mentors at UMass who helped shape this journey, Aline Gubrium, Betsy Krause, and Sonia Atalay. Thank you for your insights, your support, and your steady encouragement. I hold deep appreciation for the kinship I found among graduate students and faculty in the UMass Anthropology Department. Donna Moody (rest in power), Jon Hill, Elena Sesma, Seda Saluk, Julietta Chaparro-Buitrago, and Justin Helepololei—you all read the earliest, messiest versions of this project and offered your time, attention, and care. I am so grateful for your generosity. I am also appreciative of the American Studies faculty and my former students at Wesleyan University. That postdoctoral fellowship shaped not only some of the central questions in my thinking but also how I understand the practice of teaching itself. Those conversations, classrooms, and quiet moments of reflection left a lasting mark on the work and on me.

To my friends and colleagues at the University of Virginia: Thank you for walking alongside me in this work. In the Department of Anthropology, I am especially grateful to Jim Igoe, Sonia Alconini, Ira Bashkow, Ernesto Benítez, Eve Danziger, Lise Dobrin, Tess Farmer, Gertrude Fraser, Richard Handler, Adria LaViolette, George Mentore, Mark Sicoli, and Sylvia Tidey. In American Studies, I am indebted to Penny Von Eschen, Anna Brickhouse, Lisa Marie Cacho, Sylvia Chong, David Coyoca, Lisa Goff, Jennifer Greeson, Grace Hale, Jack Hamilton, Matt Hedstrom, Carmen Lamas, Fiona Ngô, Patricia Nguyen, and Sandhya Shukla. I'm grateful for the protection, generosity, and space you have extended to me as junior faculty and for your holding that space even more fiercely while I was on leave. Beyond my home departments, my appreciation extends to the many brilliant minds and generous colleague-friends I've had the joy of thinking with across Grounds, including the Native and

Indigenous Relations Community, the Native American Student Union, Catherine Walden, Adriana Greci-Green, Anthony Guy Lopez, Grace Softdeer, Beth Roach, Fix Cain, Teresa Pollak, Mike and Mary Wilson, and so many others whose vision and presence make this place more possible. The Black and Indigenous Feminist Futures Institute has been a space of dreaming, anchoring, and refusal. Thank you to Tiffany Lethabo King, Sonia Alconini, Lisa Cacho, Daisy Guzman Nunez, and our many brilliant collaborators for co-creating something that stretches beyond the limits of the academy. Your refusal to separate intellectual labor from embodied care has shaped how I move through this work. I'm deeply thankful as well for the administrative labor that sustains our daily worlds: Thank you to Millie Dean, Karen Hall, Bridget Murphey, Caterina Eubanks, and Brandon Block for your support, your patience, and your steady presence. And to my students: Your hard questions, deep curiosity, and refusal to settle give me hope. You carry so much of the future with you. Thank you for being brilliant, bold, and unforgiving in the best ways.

To the Choctaw people and communities in Oklahoma who trusted me with your stories, your time, and your histories, *yakoke*. You are this book's center of gravity. I am especially grateful to the *ohoyo* who welcomed me into their homes and lives and shared their stories, words, memories, and reflections with me: Thank you for your enduring generosity, insight, and clarity of purpose. To the health workers, elders, culture keepers, and youth who sat with me in clinics, kitchens, and community centers, your words reverberate far beyond these pages. I hope this work honors your refusal to disappear and your unrelenting commitment to life. To the Choctaw Nation of Oklahoma and all the people who facilitated the many moving pieces that made this research possible—from the IRB and editorial board to Food Distribution Program Director Jerry Tonubbee and the store staff across communities who let me in, answered my questions, welcomed my visits, and shared your days with me—thank you. Your openness, patience, and trust shaped every part of this project. I carry this work with a sense of responsibility that is not just scholarly but personal, rooted in kinship, in care, and in the everyday practice of honoring Choctaw sovereignty. If this book moves with any power, it is because of the relationships that made it possible, and I will remain accountable to them long after the writing ends.

In a world that often asks us to choose between joy and rigor, solitude and solidarity, I have been lucky to be in a community that insists on both and reminds me that the future we're fighting for is already being built in the ways we show up for each other. Lisa Cacho, you've supported me not just as a scholar but as a whole person, advocating for me and other junior faculty, protecting my time within the institution so I could write, mentoring me, guiding me forward, and helping me imagine my work alongside the brilliant scholars I admire. You taught me new ways to conference, how to do this work while living inside the storm of undiagnosed ADHD, and how to navigate spaces that weren't built for us. You've been there through it all—from the theoretical to the personal, from bad dates to writing breakthroughs. You opened your home to me, offered your wisdom, held my stories, thought through concepts with me, and stood beside me as a friend and colleague. You've shown me what mentorship looks like when it's infused with brilliance, honesty, loyalty, and care. You are the kind of mentor I hope to be, and if I can offer even a fraction of what you've given me to someone else, I'll consider that a success. The world is better—so much better—because you are in it. Thank you for making this ride smarter, safer, and full of joy. David Coyoca, thank you for your extraordinary generosity in sharing your gifts as a developmental editor. Your ability to read with precision and edit with clarity shaped the way I think and helped me learn how to name what I was actually trying to say. Your specialty drinks and hilarious stories have kept all of us in community. Tiffany Lethabo King, thank you for bringing BIFFI to UVA—and for bringing purpose, care, love, and scholarship to all of us along with it. Your presence has changed the landscape here, and I feel lucky to be building something alongside you. I'm as excited for the collaborative, careful work we're undertaking for liberatory futures as I am for the unfolding of our friendship. Your vision is expansive, and your way of moving through the world makes and holds space for others to breathe. Fiona Ngô and Patricia Nguyen—thank you for the gatherings, the parties, the warmth, the brilliance. Thank you for opening your home, for your hosting magic, for the joy, adventure, and care you create so effortlessly. I'm so grateful to have found scholar friends as dazzling to think with as you are fun to hang out with. You've helped make this place feel like home. To Laura Krouch, my forever best friend: You saved me over and over. You fed me, held my babies, sent funny videos, checked in on us, and kept me human. You reminded me that survival is collective, and that joy is part of the work. I miss you every day.

This project was made possible through the support of many generous funders, whose time, resources, and belief in the work allowed me to write with a little more air: the Ford Foundation; the Mellon Foundation; the Wenner-Gren Foundation; the University of Massachusetts Amherst College of Social & Behavioral Sciences; the RIDGE Center at Purdue University; the Northwest Portland Area Indian Health Board; and at the University of Virginia, the Institute of the Humanities and Global Cultures, Mapping Indigenous Worlds, Repair Lab, and Arts, Humanities, and Social Sciences Research. I am deeply grateful for this support. I am also indebted to the archivists, librarians, and community historians who safeguarded stories and guided me toward them. To those who remembered what the official records tried to forget: Your memory is resistance, and your care is its own kind of archive.

The bulk of this book was written and revised while I was a guest on the Hawaiian island of Oʻahu. When I first arrived on island, a local told me "the island chooses you." I believe this and am grateful to these lands and waters that are as beautiful and powerful as they are sacred, storied, and medicinal. Thank you for calling me in, for holding and teaching me, for loving me back, and for fostering the writing of this book. I am grateful for the life-changing friendships I've made while on the island: Heijin Lee, you are wise beyond your years, brilliant, generous, and full of life. You've taught me how to embody all the roles in my life with joy, mischief, and purpose. You remind me that we are never too old to seek wonder or fun. Brandy Nālani McDougall, my Kanaka sister who gives everything—gifts, poetry, beauty, love, grace, and story. I could listen to you for days. I love how you have a story for everything, how your warmth makes space for others to breathe, and how your generosity runs as deep as your poetry. Finally, Joyce Mariano, you are flame and refuge, a riot of laughter and joy. You showed up exactly when I needed you. Thank you for being the friend I didn't know I was missing, for seeing me when I couldn't see myself, and for becoming family without needing explanation. You kept me on track with this book, and I'll always remember our writing sessions at Talk in Kaimuki, the pages we pushed through, and the fun we always create together. I'm so grateful for the way you listen, for the clarity you bring when we talk through ideas, for reading drafts with care, and for always showing up with warmth and brilliance. Ours is a relationality rooted in joy.

To my family: Thank you for enduring the unevenness of this life. To my children, Jai and Aiona—you waited while I wrote, forgave my absences, and reminded me to return to the world. This book belongs to you as much as it does to anyone. You are the rhythm beneath the words. Amit, you began this journey with me and supported me in many ways in the writing of it. I'm grateful for the kind of parenting you give our kids— the kind I don't always know how to offer. My parents, Don and Helen: Thank you for imagining otherwise worlds, for teaching this to us even when you didn't know you were, and for being who you are, unapologetically. Your love and dreams made so many things possible. I am grateful for the ways you showed up, even when you didn't know how to stand. Mom, I found your stories after you were gone—pages tucked away, full of voice, story, hope, and magic. I know how much this book would have meant to you, even if to simply hold in your hands. I wish you could have seen it. This book carries you, too. I am lucky to have two sisters, Valarie and Meghan. I am eternally grateful that you both know the long story. We share roots, memory, and survival, and we've seen each other become and unbecome over and over. I carry you both with me everywhere. Life is no fun without you; I love you. To my grandmother, *Pokni*, Edith Aliene Gardner, *yakoke*. You storied our lives with yours; you taught us about survival, family, and humor. You carried so much more than I could ever know, and I feel you sometimes, in quiet moments and in flashes of joy. This book carries your spirit.

This book is for the ones carrying ache, longing, and fire. For those who remember what it means to be fed by land, by story, by each other. For those who refuse disappearance, who refuse to forget. For those who make kin beyond blood and who know that care is also ceremony.

COMMOD BODS

Introduction

Illness in the Everyday

Colonialism operationalizes itself, in part, by attempting to make Indigenous peoples stand in disbelief of themselves, their stories, and their histories (Watts 2013). The taking of Indigenous lands is also the attempted taking of Indigenous memories, kinship, relationalities, cosmologies, and more. Perhaps this is why so many of us begin our seemingly unfathomable stories with the caveat, "Now, I don't know how much of this is true, but. . . ." We are aware that to even hold our stories against Euro-American standards of "truth" is to accept that our stories would never fully live up to those standards (nor do we really want them to, nor should they have to), and we tell them anyway because this is how we have survived within structures that continue to attempt to eliminate us.

After the deaths of my *Pokni* (Grandma) and the other elders in our family, my dad took over the telling of our Choctaw family stories, especially the ones that we (my two sisters and I) had been too young to hear before, or that were too painful to retell, or that we had only learned to ask about as adults. My dad is an exceptional storyteller, possessing every quality of a skillful raconteur: He is imaginative, descriptive, engaging, charismatic, and theatrical, and his tales leave the listener thinking long after the story has finished. Dinners with him always include at least one story. Sometimes it's a hilarious, wild collaborative tale concocted in the very moment, and we all play along, adding to the story, largely to amuse ourselves, our children, and whoever else is present. My dad, my sisters, and I invent people and events, each of us adding another layer of fiction as everyone else listens bewildered, engaged, and asking questions in attempt to unravel the entire tale. These kinds of stories are my son's favorite memories of dinner at *Mafo's* (Grandpa's) house.

My dad's storytelling—especially when it turns toward painful stories—follows a familiar ritual. It almost always begins post-meal, after he's opened a second bottle of heavy, overpriced wine and poured it, mostly for himself and his partner. The wine is not incidental. It's what makes the telling possible, loosening memory, muting shame, perhaps allowing him to feel without completely unraveling. It is both a condition of possibility for these particular stories to be told and a response to them. This ritual—post-meal, glasses full, his voice slowing and growing solemn—creates an atmosphere that my sisters and I recognize instantly. We exchange glances across the table, bracing ourselves. As his face flushes and his eyes grow glassy, he begins: "Now, listen to this." What follows is not just a narrative but an engagement with something much deeper: a transmission of memory and grief, shaped by the emotional residues of intergenerational trauma. These aren't just family stories; they're embedded within what Billy-Ray Belcourt (2018) calls "the exhausted existence of indigeneity," a state marked by "the miserable feeling of not properly being of this world." In those moments, my dad inhabits that exhaustion. The act of storytelling becomes a form of endurance. It is an attempt to make sense of the senseless, an effort to pass down pain without drowning in it, and a lived expression of the ongoingness of colonial violence. And we, his daughters, sit in that with him, listening and remembering. The stories matter, but so do the conditions under which they're told, marking both a refusal to forget and a struggle to survive the remembrance. On one such occasion years ago, my dad elaborated on Pokni's life post-boarding school, telling us something she had never shared with us when we all lived together. Pokni had always been open about her time at Chilocco Indian Agricultural School,[1] the Indian boarding school she and Annie[2] attended. Located about 225 miles from their home and known for its highly structured and strict military regime, it completely devastated Pokni and Annie. Her stories were tempered for our young ages, and while she didn't share the grainy details with us, her granddaughters, we knew that she and Annie had lived in constant fear.

They were forbidden to speak *Chahta anumpa* (the Choctaw language), suffered through threats of separation from each other, and were isolated from the rest of their family. They attempted to run away from Chilocco on multiple occasions, sneaking out in the middle of the night, carrying handkerchiefs stuffed with food bits they had secretly stashed, planning to walk all the way home—for however long it would take, no matter how dangerous it was—because the alternative (remaining at Chilocco) was unbearable. After each escape, however, they were caught and brought back to the school. Each time, they suffered the consequences. But this time at the dinner table, my dad shared with us what had happened after Pokni and Annie had finally made it out of Chilocco.

According to my dad, when they returned home after three years at the school, their lives were completely different. Their parents had died; a white family was living in their house and had taken over their land; and they could not immediately locate any living family members. Their entire world had been erased. Pokni and Annie eventually found one of their cousins, Anakfi, at a hospital more than two hundred miles north. When they visited him, he was highly medicated and able to tell them only bits and pieces of what had happened: When their father died, he left Anakfi the family's property and wealth.[3] Shortly thereafter, a local judge trespassed on their land. Anakfi fired a warning shot at him, and the next day he was taken in for "shooting at a judge." Things moved very swiftly after that: Anakfi was arrested, declared insane, and locked up in an "insane asylum" in the northeast corner of the state. No other beneficiaries for the family's estate were identified, and everything went to the judge as compensation. It was the judge's family that Pokni and Annie saw living in their family home when they returned from Chilocco. Having nothing else, they made their way to Tulsa, got jobs together in a meatpacking factory, and built a new world for themselves in the city. As adults, Pokni and Annie both lived very difficult lives filled with instability, violence, and oppression, and they suffered greatly from preventable (or at least treatable) health problems. Furthermore, their children, my father and two uncles, have all been beset by alcoholism, shame, grief, and a consuming sadness.

This is the story my dad shared with us, as he had been told it and as he remembered. I don't know how much of it is "true," so I share it with trepidation, but I share it nonetheless because it is the story my dad tells, stands by, and has become one of our family's narratives. It is not thoroughly researched or backed up with paperwork; I have not done my due diligence to check the accuracy of the details. In fact, I struggle to talk about some of our family stories because I don't trust that they're completely true. As an example, my dad loved telling a particular story about the extravagant wealth of some of our Choctaw ancestors—one uncle who had a car was so wealthy that when the car ran out of gas, he just left it on the side of the road and bought a new car. I found this an unbelievable story, something grandiose that reflected my dad's particular desire to live outside of poverty and claim roots to something ridiculously lavish (because anyone who knows my dad knows he is like this). When I was in graduate school, though, my professor asked us to share a family story as part of an exercise in critically interrogating memory. That story came back to me, and I decided to investigate its possibility. It turns out that abandoning cars in rural Oklahoma during the early days of automobiles was a real thing because the infrastructure for gasoline stations did not exist. In that moment, I am embarrassed to admit, I began to reconsider not only the truthfulness of some of our family stories, but to also critically reflect on and believe in the purpose of the stories—the meaning-making, the important work that the stories *do*—and to trust the storyteller. To trust the storyteller and the stories is to trust that the stories are living, mutable, and evolving teachings, lessons, and values being transmitted and shared at particular moments for particular reasons, and they are legible in different ways for different listeners. As listeners, it is our responsibility to make sense of the stories, to take what speaks to us seriously, and to learn.

This is not a project about the accuracy of Choctaw oral stories, or about fact-checking family lore and handed-down tales. Those are important endeavors for lots of reasons and matter to many people with varying agendas, but this project is interested in the kind of work the stories *do*: Which stories are shared, when, and for whom? *Who* is doing the telling, *why* are they telling these stories, *how* are they telling these stories? *Why* are they important, meaningful, and selected to be shared, continuing across generations? *What* do these stories accomplish? And *how* do these stories affect health, specifically Indigenous health experiences, outcomes, and medical narratives? In asking these questions, I began to understand that my dad, like so many other Native people of his generation, share these stories—in part—to make sense of what they are experiencing today and to share something close to a set of instructions for us and for the future. It is these spaces of meaning-making that I argue provide a theoretical framework for understanding the linkages between historical trauma and its manifestation in health outcomes among Indigenous peoples.

I grew up witnessing and experiencing my family's struggles with all sorts of socio-economic and health-related problems, and I grew up in Native communities in Oklahoma where lots of people were going through similar experiences. I came to understand that diabetes, alcoholism, and premature, unjust morbidity and mortality seemed to be a regular part of life. It was only later in life that I realized these experiences are indeed a regular part of life, but only for *some* of us. I entered graduate school to understand this exact question. Making sense of my family's terrible health problems and stories—stories that are not unique among Indigenous people—became my focus. I wanted to use the lens of anthropology to understand the linkages between historical trauma and its manifestation in health outcomes. As I talked with tribal citizens across rural, southeastern Oklahoma and the urban centers of Tulsa and Oklahoma City, obesity surfaced as an identifiable, problematic, and major health concern for Choctaws. Elders, key community leaders, and tribal citizens employed as Choctaw Nation service providers (e.g., social workers, program coordinators, staff members, etc.) pointed to obesity and its related chronic health problems—specifically diabetes and, to a lesser degree, heart disease—as the biggest health outcomes concerns in their communities. Surprisingly, several of the people I spoke with knew the stark statistics of obesity among Oklahoma Indians,[4] and others informed me about obesity prevention programs they were aware of, both through the Choctaw Nation of Oklahoma (CNO) and in connection with the state health department and local universities. Their concerns about obesity stemmed from their knowledge of the obesity-related health conditions (i.e., diabetes and related outcomes such as amputations, blindness, dialysis, and heart disease) that they saw, experienced, and helped to manage among their friends, family members, and selves.

The summer after the first year in my PhD program, I traveled around the greater areas of Tulsa and Oklahoma City and across communities within the borders of the CNO in the south-eastern part of the state, specifically Broken Bow, Durant, McAlester, and Poteau. Many of the people I met with spoke about obesity in more complex ways than simply statistical indicators of health. They talked about obesity (or large bodies, largeness, or fatness) as a social connector, a marker of Indianness, describing being "skinny" as akin to being "white." People also tied in foods like fry bread, Indian tacos, and other contemporary foodstuffs as traditional Choctaw foods that contributed to fat bodies and poor health. They also linked obesity with commodity foods, or participation in the Food Distribution Program on Indian Reservations (FDPIR), joking about "commod bods," or bodies made fat from the consumption of commodity foods high in fat and calories. This early exploratory fieldwork across Oklahoma and within Choctaw communities mapped out the direction of my larger research question—in what ways is historical trauma linked with poor health outcomes?—inspiring me to examine broadly the historical, socio-political, economic, and cultural forces that have made possible the conditions for obesity, for fat bodies to be seen as *Indian* bodies. Specifically, this project became tasked with examining the trifecta of FDPIR participation, poverty, and processes of cultural identity to understand how and in what ways these associations materialize into obesity among Choctaws.

While my family's story may seem extreme, it sadly shares many commonalities with the majority of the women's stories included in this project. Ninety percent of these women revealed trauma experiences—historical or generational trauma and/or structural violence—in their food-centered life history narratives. At the time of this research, which was conducted between 2013 and 2016, most women (85 percent) were clinically classified as either overweight (22 percent) or obese (63 percent), and more than half (60 percent) suffered from type 2 diabetes. Scholars have employed constructs of historical trauma to describe the impacts and legacies of colonization, cultural and material dispossession, and historical oppression in relation to health outcomes (Braveheart and DeBruyn 1998; Evans-Campbell 2008; Gone 2014; Sotero 2006). Specific to obesity, scholarship points to historical trauma as a contributing factor that shapes all other factors, linking environmental obesogenic conditions with centuries-old colonization practices and assimilation policies that dispossessed people of their lands and undermined their opportunities to live empowered lives (Sotero 2006; Willows et al. 2012). Historical and ongoing practices and policies (e.g., boarding schools, forced removals, bans on traditional fishing and hunting practices, and water restrictions) contribute to impoverished foodscapes (Winson 2004) and loss of traditional ways that disrupt the transference of parenting, life skills, and knowledge (Sotero 2006; Willows et al. 2012). Researchers now advocate for the inclusion of a historical perspective to obesity prevention in Indian communities, one that contextualizes the influences of colonization and social inequities on weight status, including prenatal, sociocultural, family, and community environments.

This book provides a narrative window into the ways in which Choctaw women make sense of their experiences of obesity and related conditions in southeastern Oklahoma. I determine such experiences to be interlinked with the ways in which historical trauma is a public collective, which these women call upon to make sense of their present experiences of inequality and poor health. I use the construct of historical trauma as *public narrative* (Mohatt et al. 2014) to understand the ways in which meaning-making occurs, as opposed to a biomedical approach that considers obesity (and diabetes) a disease largely detached from social contexts, and especially meaning-making. I am further interested in the ways in which historical trauma is used as an explanation of obesity and how that interacts with the macro-level forces of history, political economy, and contemporary forms of violence, as well as heritage narratives evoked to underpin individual and group identity. Examining obesity at these intersections provides a good case to analyze how disparate health outcomes among Choctaws, and Indigenous peoples in North America more generally, are historically situated, socially driven, understood as co-constructed, and made sense of in profound ways.

I have coined the term *embodied heritage* to illustrate the key components that I found to be fundamental for understanding the health and well-being of overweight and obese Choctaw women in the Choctaw Nation. The first component includes historical trauma and the ways it is called upon as public narrative to account for and make sense of contemporary health disparities and social ills. The second component is violence and encompasses structural, symbolic, and everyday forms of violence. The third component includes heritage, which is defined here as the active process of remembering that underpins identity and the ways in which people make sense of their experiences in the present

(Smith 2006). The fourth component is identity, particularly the social production of Indian identity through obesity. The final component (specific to this book) is obesity (or overweight)—the women in this study are connected through their shared "fatness" (only five women fell into a "normal" body mass index category). The first four components of embodied heritage are interconnected and inseparable from each other (dialectical and even porous), thus providing a deeper understanding of the fifth component (obesity). Embodied heritage, then, focuses on meaning-making, personal and public narratives, and cultural identities. Put simply, an embodied heritage framework posits that health is contingent on one's social, economic, historical, cultural, and political position *and* on the structures of meaning that make sense of this personal and embodied experience.

In this book, I situate the embodied heritage framework within Native American Indigenous studies, yet it is informed significantly by the field of critical biocultural anthropology. The introduction begins with a brief overview of the influence of political economy on health. With a focus on critical biocultural anthropology, I define the contemporary forms of violence that play a central role in women's narratives and connect these with historical trauma. Second, I describe the emergence of obesity as a major health concern within the United States and among Native Americans specifically and examine the historical dependence on government-supplied foods, with a focus on the Choctaw Nation of Oklahoma. Third, I introduce the biocultural dimensions of obesity among Choctaws, describing the structural and social forces that contribute to obesity. Finally, I describe the embodied heritage construct in depth, discuss why this approach is useful, and ground it with the example of "commod bod" that arose early in my fieldwork. After this theoretical orientation, I provide an overview of the subsequent chapters.

The Political Economy of Health

A central goal of critical biocultural anthropology is understanding the complexities of the causes and consequences of health, illness, and social well-being among vulnerable groups, including the power relations that structure social inequalities. In this section, I introduce theory from critical biocultural and medical anthropology that shapes my understanding of the ways in which political-economic and social inequalities facilitate individualized suffering and disease among the poor, using my family's story as a stepping-off point.

Critical biocultural and medical anthropologists have emphasized violence—both overt and covert—as a significant factor contributing to health inequality (Dressler 2005; Farmer 1996; Goodman and Leatherman 1998; Kleinman 1997, 2000; Leatherman 2005; Leatherman and Goodman 2011; Rylko-Bauer et al. 2009; Scheper-Hughes and Bourgois 2004; Singer and Hodge 2010). The impact and consequences of visible violence, such as that experienced during wars and conflicts, is readily apparent on the health of those affected; however, the enduring effects of invisible violence, like my grandmother's experiences of boarding school or experiences of food insecurity and poverty, are more difficult to measure and often manifest only months or years later.

Anthropological literature extensively explores three primary modes of violence: structural, symbolic, and everyday violence, each of which provides critical insights into understanding health disparities such as obesity, particularly among Native American communities. These forms of violence do not operate in isolation; rather, they are deeply interconnected, reinforcing and intensifying their collective impact. Additionally, they are entangled with historical trauma, shaping social and health outcomes in profound and often insidious ways. By analyzing each mode separately, while acknowledging their interdependence, we can better grasp how they shape individual and collective experiences, influencing identity, health, and well-being.

The concept of *structural violence* originated primarily from the field of sociology, particularly the work of Johan Galtung, a Norwegian sociologist who introduced the term in 1969 to describe how systemic social structures and institutions harm or disadvantage people by restricting their ability to meet basic needs. Structural violence operates through deeply embedded inequalities within institutions, policies, and economic systems, making it an essential framework for understanding how hidden mechanisms perpetuate disparities in health, wealth, and opportunity (Bourgois 2001, 2009; Farmer 1999; Farmer et al. 2006). Anthropologist Nancy Scheper-Hughes (2004:13) defines *structural violence* as the "invisible social machinery of inequality," a mechanism that reproduces exclusion and marginalization through ideologies, stigmas, and discourses that make poverty, hunger, and illness appear natural or inevitable. These inequalities are rarely attributed to their structural roots; instead, blame is often placed on the individuals suffering from them. As Paul Farmer (1992, 2004) notes, structural violence is embodied as disease, oppression, and even genocide, creating a feedback loop of disadvantage.

For my grandmother, the political and ideological structures that facilitated policies of Indian removal and assimilation forced her to attend boarding schools and fueled the dismantling of her family, culture, and materiality. Breaking families apart shaped the lack of accountability provided by social networks, which made possible the swift and uncontested stealing of Choctaw property,[5] leading to material dispossession and a weakened collectivity that might have otherwise provided resistance to dispossession. This particular form of violence, the severing of intergenerational knowledge and community cohesion through institutionalized subjugation, was central to the narratives of many Choctaw women I spoke with as they reflected on the ways colonial policies shaped their families, foodways, and health outcomes.

French sociologist Pierre Bourdieu introduced the concept of *symbolic violence* (1989, 2001), which refers to the subtle, often invisible ways that dominant social groups impose their norms, values, and beliefs on marginalized groups, making social hierarchies appear natural and unquestionable. Unlike direct physical violence, symbolic violence operates through internalized social expectations, shaping how individuals perceive themselves and their place in society. Symbolic violence is enacted through language, cultural representations, and social expectations, reinforcing power structures in ways that seem inevitable or self-imposed (Bourdieu and Wacquant 1992). This form of violence is particularly insidious because it influences marginalized individuals to adopt the very ideologies that oppress them. Bourdieu and Wacquant (2004:273) argue that symbolic violence includes "the domination of the dominant by his domination," meaning that the oppressed are often compelled to conform to the very standards that exclude them.

In my fieldwork, this was particularly evident in how Choctaw women spoke about obesity and food choices. Some interlocutors described obesity and unhealthy eating patterns as markers of Indianness, reinforcing racialized narratives that link Native identity to struggle, poverty, and poor health. This reflects a broader dynamic in which Indigenous peoples are held to impossible standards of authenticity, expected to maintain a cultural continuity that colonial violence has actively disrupted (Barker 2011; Povinelli 2002). When traditional practices become inaccessible (for multiple reasons), symbolic violence fills the gap by shaping alternative identities that conform to social expectations, even when those identities are harmful. For example, fat Indigenous bodies are often portrayed in public health and media discourse as symbols of dysfunction, reinforcing the idea that Indigenous people are "bad at life" (Belcourt 2018). This narrative naturalizes health disparities as a self-inflicted failure rather than the product of historical and structural oppression. By examining symbolic violence, we can better understand how Indigenous identity is continuously negotiated in the face of external pressures and how these pressures influence perceptions of health, food, and self-worth.

Finally, *everyday violence*, as conceptualized by Scheper-Hughes (1992) and Bourgois (1998, 2004, 2009), refers to the routine, normalized acts of violence that become so embedded in daily life that they are no longer recognized as violence at all. While structural violence is tied to systemic inequalities, and symbolic violence operates through internalized social hierarchies, everyday violence manifests in repeated, routine encounters that reinforce oppression and marginalization. In the communities where I conducted research, race-based everyday violence was frequently experienced through public displays of Native caricature and stereotype. For example, in Broken Bow, Oklahoma, home to the highest density of Choctaws in the state, the local high school football team is called the "Broken Bow Savages." The school's mascot is

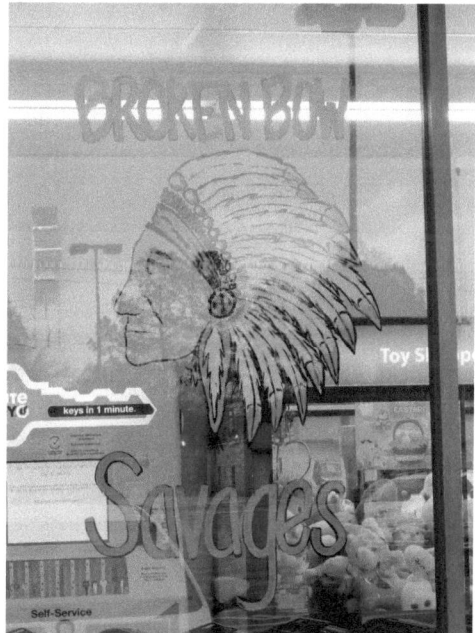

FIGURE 1 Broken Bow Savages High School mascot. Photo by Kasey Jernigan (author).

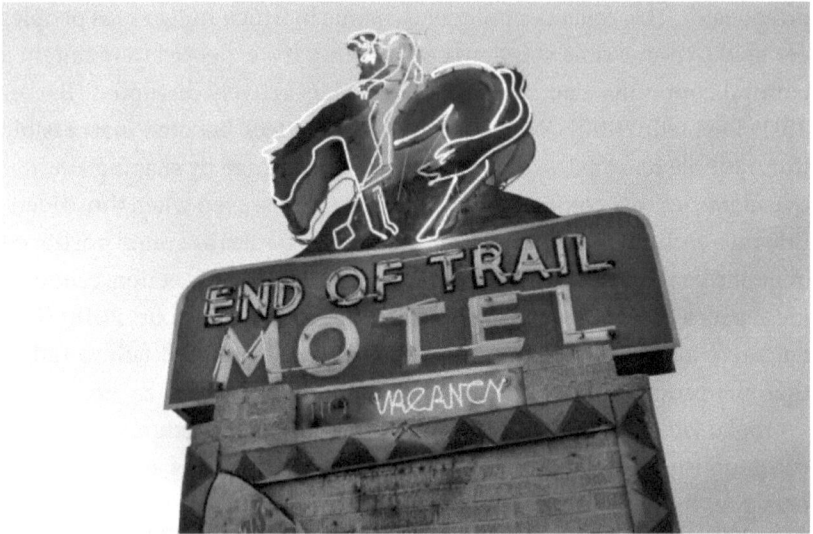

FIGURE 2 End of Trail Motel. Photo by Clayton Fraser.

a stereotypical depiction of a Native person in a headdress, displayed prominently on the school's walls, sports fields, and even a local Wal-Mart. Similarly, the End of Trail Motel, a dilapidated structure at the main intersection of the town, signals both a literal and figurative narrative of Indigenous erasure. These symbols of Native caricature are not passive representations; they actively participate in the everyday violence of racialization. They create an environment where Indigenous peoples are reminded (constantly, pervasively) that their identities are subject to mockery, commodification, and erasure. The existence of Native mascots and harmful stereotypes does more than offend; it contributes to inter-generational trauma by reinforcing narratives of inferiority, Otherness, and cultural death.

Everyday violence also shapes access to health and well-being. The stigma surrounding Native health disparities, particularly obesity and diabetes, creates environments where Indigenous individuals face blame rather than support. Public health institutions and media narratives of-ten present Native bodies as inherently unhealthy, obscuring the role of colonial violence in shaping contemporary food systems and access to nutrition. As a result, many Indigenous individuals experience routine microaggressions in medical settings, workplaces, and public spaces, reinforcing their marginalization and limiting their ability to seek care without judgment.

Understanding these three forms of violence—structural, symbolic, and everyday—as interconnected forces is essential for analyzing health disparities in Indigenous communities and frames my analysis of the social and political-economic inequities and individualized trauma and subjugation that contribute to poor health outcomes among Natives and among the women in my study in particular. Yet, these forms of violence cannot be disconnected from historical trauma (i.e., widespread injustices experienced by Indigenous peoples that span generations), and indeed this connection has long been overlooked. The greatest source of historical trauma, rooted in systemic genocidal violence, may be the displacement of people from their homelands and assimilation practices to "kill the Indian." The loss of one's connection to family and cultural identity through land alienation has been strongly associated with poor health outcomes. As Peña notes, "place-breaking makes heart-breaking possible" (2011:209).

Obesity Trends

The World Health Organization has declared obesity a global epidemic, and in 2000 it was estimated that, for the first time in history, there were more overweight than underweight people globally (Anderson et al. 2009; Bell et al. 2017; Brewis 2011; Brockett 1990). In the United States, the latest National Health and Nutrition Examination Survey (NHANES)[6] data show the adult obesity rate between 2017 and 2020 is nearly 42 percent (a 37 percent increase from 1999–2000), and the national youth obesity rate is nearly 20 percent (a 42 percent increase for the same timeframes) (Emmerich et al. 2023). Another way of considering the drastic increase of obesity in the United States is to compare the number of states with adult obesity rates at or above 35 percent over time: In 1985, no state had an adult obesity rate higher than 15 percent; in 1991, no state was over 20 percent; in 2000, no state was over 25 percent; and in 2006, only Mississippi and West Virginia were above 30 percent.

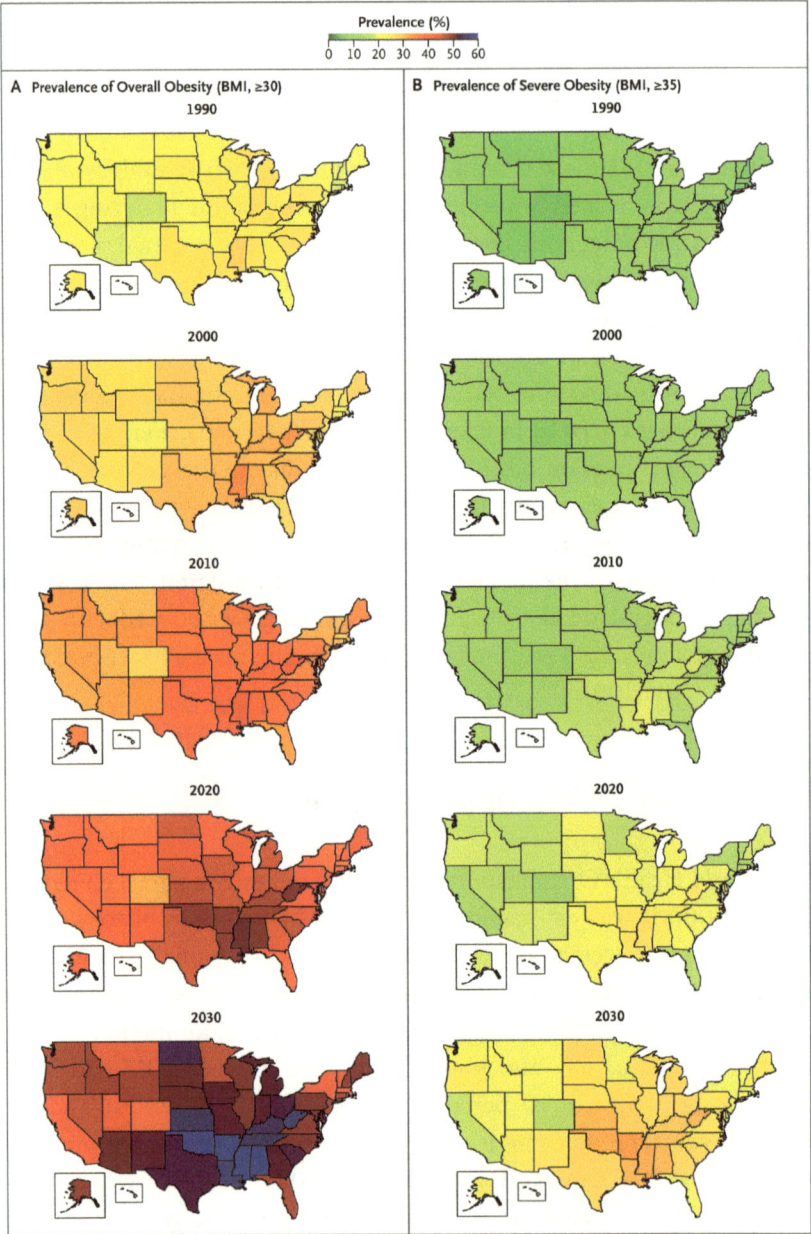

FIGURE 3 Estimated prevalence of overall obesity and severe obesity in each state. Shown is the estimated prevalence of overall obesity (Panel A) and severe obesity (Panel B) among adults in each U.S. state from 1990 through 2030. Overall obesity includes the BMI (body-mass index) categories of moderate obesity (BMI of 30 to < 35) and severe obesity (BMI of ≥ 35). Courtesy of Ward et al., 2019.

In 2022, twenty-two states had obesity rates at or above 35 percent, and three states—Louisiana, Oklahoma, and West Virginia—had an obesity prevalence of 40 percent or greater (CDC, 2023).

Long-term trends predict that by 2030, nearly one in two adults will have obesity, with prevalence rates higher than 50 percent in twenty-nine states and not below 35 percent in *any* state. Nearly one in every four adults is projected to have severe obesity by 2030, with data showing that severe obesity is likely to become the most common body mass index (BMI) category among women, non-Hispanic Black adults, and low-income adults (Ward et al. 2019). American Indians/Alaska Natives (AI/AN)[7] are 50 percent more likely to have obesity than non-Hispanic whites, with 48.1 percent of AI/AN adults having obesity (CDC 2023). Furthermore, AI/AN women are 70 percent more likely than white women to have obesity (Barnes et al. 2011), and among AI/AN children and adolescents, obesity is more than two times more common than among non-Hispanic white (16 percent) or Asian (13 percent) youth (Anderson and Whitaker, 2009; Ogden et al. 2010).

Currently the ninth most obese state in the U.S., data predict Oklahoma will become the most obese state by 2030. The 2022 Oklahoma State Department of Health Obesity Prevention Plan Report (OSDH 2022) declares that as of 2019, one million Oklahoma adults have obesity—in other words, one out of every three adults, with some counties in the state reporting more than 50 percent of the adult population having obesity. Figure 4 shows that in the Choctaw Nation, located in the southeastern part of the state, obesity prevalence ranges from 32 percent to 53 percent. OSDH (2022) data show that more than 50 percent of adult AIs in Oklahoma have obesity (compared with 38 percent of non-Hispanic white adults), and 17 percent of Oklahoma AIs have been diagnosed with type 2 diabetes (compared with 12 percent of non-Hispanic whites in Oklahoma).[8]

Why is obesity considered such an important health concern? From public health and medical perspectives, obesity is linked with a range of physical and mental conditions at the population level, leading to increased healthcare expenses and losses in productivity. Research shows that adults with obesity face an elevated risk of numerous diseases, including type 2 diabetes, hypertension, cardiovascular disease, stroke, arthritis, depression, sleep apnea, liver and kidney disease, gallbladder disease, pregnancy-related issues, various cancers, and more recently severe complications from COVID-19 (Angelantonio et al. 2016; Flegal and Kalantar-Zadeh 2013; Greenberg 2013; Kompaniyets 2021; Lauby-Secretan et al. 2016; Leddy et al. 2008; NIDDK 2023; NIH Obesity Education Initiative Expert Panel 1998). Adults with obesity have a higher overall risk of mortality. Among children with obesity, the risks are similar, with the addition that such children are more likely to have obesity as adults. The medical costs for individuals with obesity are higher when compared to those of lower-weight individuals. A 2021 study revealed that obesity added $170 billion to annual medical expenses in the United States (Ward et al. 2021). Additionally, the indirect costs of obesity, such as missed school and workdays, reduced productivity, premature death, and higher transportation costs, also amount to billions of dollars (Hammond and Levine 2010; Harris and Werman 2014; Wang et al. 2015).

In 2010, the Choctaw Nation opened a Diabetes Wellness Center, emphasizing its commitment to the treatment and prevention of obesity and diabetes. This commitment was also reiterated in then-Chief Gregory Pyle's 2010 State of the Nation's Health Report, which launched the tribe's Going Lean Initiative. This was directed by a community advisory board consisting of tribal leaders, elders, health planners, and policy makers, with the goal of reducing and preventing obesity (*Native American Times* 2011; Schorow 2010). The first two years of the initiative focused on individual-level health promotion efforts, including exercise, healthy cooking classes, and lifestyle or motivational counseling. The Going Lean Team's main focus is on obesity prevention and promoting healthy lifestyles. Today, Going Lean has more than 3,000 active members[9] in the Promoting Active Communities Everywhere (PACE) program which, to remain an active member, demands participation in an event (a 5K, 10K, 15K, or half-marathon) every six months. Going Lean also hosts fitness and cultural camps for youth ages nine to eleven, with about one hundred youth participating in the three day/two night-camp annually.

Clearly missing from the Going Lean initiative is a greater understanding of how Choctaws (and other residents in the CNO) biologically incorporate their lived experiences, thereby creating these particular population patterns of health and disease that, in turn, reflect the connections between bodies and the body politic; in other words, the embodiment of obesity. This cannot be understood without reference to historical processes and to individual and social modes of living, as well as to larger forces of the political economy (Krieger 2001; Yamada & Palmer 2006). Nor can we understand obesity among Indigenous peoples without also including Indigenous understandings of obesity which, like non-Indigenous populations, are multi-factorial but unique in relational aspects and connectedness to each other and the environment, as determinants for obesity expression (Bell et al. 2017). As Krieger (2005:350) writes, "bodies tell stories about—and cannot be studied divorced from—the conditions of our existence."

Historical Context

Indigenous foodways have historically been unique to local ecosystems, based largely on a collective understanding and awareness of local environments, and grounded in principles of balance and interconnectedness (Graesch et al. 2010; VanDerwarker et al. 2013). Choctaws, originally from the southeastern part of the United States, cultivated maize, beans, and squash; hunted deer, wild turkey, and small game; and harvested local edibles. These foodways were largely disrupted during Indian removal between 1829 and 1831, when Choctaws were relocated to unfamiliar land in Indian Territory (present-day Oklahoma) (Bodirsky and Johnson 2008; Briggs 2015; Vantrease 2013; Wiedman 2012). During this time, the U.S. government implemented a policy to make farmers out of all North American Indians, with the ultimate goal of their assimilation into white society (Banner 2009; Hurt 1987; Robertson 2005). To prevent starvation during this transition to self-sufficient farming in new lands, as well as part of treaty agreements for forced removal, the government provided temporary rations to tribes (Mailer and Hale 2015; Mihesuah 2016; Wiedman 2012). Anthropologist Dennis Wiedman (2012) provides an early example of the kinds of rations provided in 1869 to tribes in Oklahoma, which included beef, bacon, flour, corn meal, coffee, salt, and sugar. The rations, which were intended to prevent starvation rather than emphasize nutrition, were heavily processed and preserved to endure the long journeys to their destinations. Wiedman's (2012) review of foods and goods distributed to Oklahoma reservations in the late 1800s identifies the bureaucratic standardization and routinization of foods and goods by the Office of Indian Affairs, making visible how the U.S. government has long played a significant role in (re)shaping the food environments of Indigenous peoples (see also Joe and Young 1994; Mihesuah 2016; Milburn 2004).

Today, the U.S. Department of Agriculture's (USDA) Food Distribution Program on Indian Reservations (FDPIR) supplies a monthly food package program to nearly 100,000 people in approximately 275 tribes, including the Choctaw Nation of Oklahoma (USDA 2014). This program began in the 1960s in response to severe and widespread poverty, malnutrition, and hunger; by the 1970s, Indian communities were consuming mostly government-provided commodities. This pattern largely continues today, with around 60 percent of rural and reservation Indians and 20 percent of urban Indians relying on commodity foods as their primary food source (Dillinger 1999; Halpern 2007). Studies show that regular and continued use of commodity foods over the life course influences food use and food preference (Chino and DeBruyn 2006; Dillinger 1999). Included in the FDPIR today are canned foods such as meats, beans, vegetables, soups, and fruits; bottled juices; cereals; rice; dried pasta; flours; processed cheese; powdered egg mix; shelf-stable milk; buttery spread; and vegetable oil. The resemblance to the early rations of the 1800s is clear: Many of today's commodity foods are heavily preserved, shelf-stable, have a low nutritional value, continue to be supplied by the government, and have forced adoption of new foods and practices. Tribal governments recognize this and have recently made fresh fruits, vegetables, and select meats available, but because these foods are part of a federal package, they remain non-localized, consist of surplus foods, and are still transported long distances.

The FDPIR officially began in the CNO in 1984, and families originally lined up outside a tractor-trailer truck to receive their monthly bulk food package. Today, the Choctaw Nation has five Food Distribution locations across its reservation. These locations offer grocery store-style distribution, with aisles and scanners. Rather than receiving a monthly box of foods, families may now come as frequently as needed to obtain foods. A recent addition is the purchase of a bobtail truck and frozen trailer that assists in transporting frozen meats and goods to families who live a considerable distance from the nearest distribution location. Currently, 5,000–6,000 individuals (2,500–3,000 households) per month participate in the Food Distribution Program in the Choctaw Nation (Hutto 2017).

Participation in food and nutrition assistance programs, including the FDPIR, has been shown to significantly elevate the risk of obesity, particularly among women (Adams et al. 2003; Gibson 2003; Martin and Ferris 2007; Townsend et al. 2001), and the unhealthy food preferences now prevalent among Native Americans have been attributed to FDPIR (Dillinger 1999). Scholars argue that food plays a major part of cultural survival and affirmation (Bisogni et al. 2002; Counihan 2002); thus, the demise of traditional Indigenous foodways *should* signify cultural extinction. Yet, we see Indigenous peoples in the United States linking colonial experiences of FDPIR participation (i.e., commodity foods) with loss of land and food sovereignty, thus invoking shared and collective experiences of injustice that inform contemporary cultural identities (Maxwell 2014; Roy 2006; Saerth 2010; Vantrease 2013). In other words, instead of signifying cultural extinction, the demise of traditional foodways is recognized as a specific experience that informs what it means to be Indigenous today. For example, the term "commod bod" that arose in my early fieldwork is commonly used in Native communities (and especially in urban communities) to refer to the body type that results from consuming commodity foods high in fat and calories. Although used humorously, "commod bod" serves as a marker for Indianness identified by poor food environments, dependence on food assistance, and obesity. When a group is marginalized by race, ethnicity, language, or religion, food often takes on distinct meaning as a vehicle for transmitting cultural traditions and identities. FDPIR foods, or commodity foods, have become locally known as "Indian food," thus providing an understudied lens of cultural survival mediated through food.

Biocultural Dimensions of Obesity

Embodiment refers to how we biologically incorporate our lived experiences, or how social influences impact the physical body (Lock and Farquhar 2007; Mascia-Lees 2011), and is a useful framework for assessing health disparities because it explores biosocial relationships (Krieger 2005). Pathways to embodiment are multiple, occur at multiple levels, and are often structured by 1) arrangements of power, property, production, consumption, and reproduction; and 2) human biology as it is shaped by evolution, ecology, and individual life histories (Krieger 2001, 2005; Yamada and Palmer 2006).

Arrangements of Power, Property, Production, Consumption, and Reproduction

Food insecurity exists when the availability of nutritionally adequate and safe foods, or the ability to acquire acceptable foods in socially acceptable ways, is limited or uncertain (Willows et al. 2012). Food insecurity also includes the fear of not being able to provide or obtain food (Anderson 1990).[10] The food insecurity rate of Oklahoma is 17 percent, the highest in the nation,[11] and the two counties with the highest food insecurity are within the CNO boundaries: Choctaw County (21 percent food insecure) and McCurtain County (24 percent food insecure) (Hake et al. 2024).

Approximately 20 percent of Choctaws living in the Choctaw Nation participate in the FDPIR, and most report using commodity foods for at least one meal per day, mainly due to limited access to grocery stores (CNO 2012). Among those who do live in closer proximity to a grocery store, most elect to drive longer distances, usually monthly, to do bulk shopping at Wal-Mart Supercenters for more variety and better-quality produce at significantly lower prices than at the smaller local grocery stores. Additionally, tribal members report shopping at one of the thirteen tribally owned convenience stores at least weekly for both snacks and meals. All of these convenience stores serve fresh, prepared, and packaged foods, primarily high in fat and sugar, and several of the stores have mini casinos and seating areas.

Demographic and socioeconomic conditions constrain the food choices that families make. Families are important social environments that shape health, diet, and practices related to physical activities for children (Hill and Lissau 2006), so practices related to food acquisition, preparation, and eating habits for families in the Choctaw Nation are important sites to consider. Among families with limited resources, emphasis is often on selecting foods that family members will eat rather than attempting to introduce new foods that may go to waste. Additionally, historical trauma offers explanations of poor diet and physical inactivity by linking abrupt and forced removal from families, broken bonds between parents and children, and disrupted transference of parenting skills (Willows et al. 2012).

Pathways to embodiment of obesity among Choctaws also include the environment, namely the rurality of the reservation as it contributes to the determinants of physical activity, including sedentary lifestyles. Towns within the reservation lack walkable neighborhoods or safe, available, and accessible parks or recreation areas. They are made up of sprawling countryside with long distances to tribal wellness centers, and the extreme weather[12] in southeastern Oklahoma can often limit outdoor activity. Moreover, the limited number of grocery stores and multiple fast-food establishments help to determine the foodscape across the reservation (Winson 2004:301). Communities with fewer supermarkets and more fast food and convenience stores have higher rates of obesity (Laraia et al. 2004; Lee 2012; Sallis and Glanz 2006). A study in Washington state found that reservations had fewer available, and more costly, fresh vegetables and fruits compared to non-reservation communities nearby (O'Connell et al. 2011); other studies report that in lieu of supermarkets, many Native Americans purchase foods from convenience stores (McKinnon et al. 2009; Pareo-Tubbeh et al. 2000). Conversations with women in this project indicate that this is true for Choctaws as well.

Human Biology as Shaped by Evolution, Ecology, and Life Histories

High birth weights among Indigenous peoples have been observed over several decades and across several regions in the United States and Canada. A woman's weight status in pregnancy influences the future weight status of her offspring and their risk for type 2 diabetes (Bloomgarden 2010; Herring and Oken 2011; Rasmussen 2009). Limited information is available regarding factors associated with Native birth weight or infant growth patterns, with the majority of research dedicated to maternal diabetes status (either diabetes pre-pregnancy or gestational diabetes mellitus). Research indicates that children of women with previous gestational diabetes have an increased risk of developing childhood obesity, pre-diabetes, and type 2 diabetes (Bellamy 2009). A Danish study found that by nineteen to twenty-seven years of age, these children had an eight-fold

risk of prediabetes or diabetes (Damm 2009). Among Natives in Oklahoma, the prevalence of gestational diabetes is 12 percent (compared to
9 percent of non-Hispanic whites in Oklahoma) (OSDH, 2012).

Infant feeding practices influence both the rate of infant growth and
body fat accumulation, with research linking longer breastfeeding du-
ration with a lower risk of pediatric overweight (Willows et al. 2012). A
study of Indigenous children who were exclusively breastfed for longer
than twelve weeks (compared with less than or equal to twelve weeks)
showed a significant inverse association with overweight at age eight to
ten years (Mai et al. 2007). The Centers for Disease Control estimates
that, for every month a child is breastfed, the child's risk for childhood
overweight decreases by 4 percent, plateauing at nine months of age
(Yan et al. 2014). Oklahoma Natives have the lowest percentage of all
"races" for breastfeeding (15 percent for six months or more compared
to 31 percent for non-Hispanic whites) (OSDH 2011). Women, Infants,
and Children data for 2023 indicate that in the Choctaw Nation, only
11 percent of infants were fully breastfed, and nearly 80 percent were
fully formula-fed (USDA 2023). Conversations with women in this
project reveal that infant breastfeeding practices and attitudes are
strongly influenced by broken bonds between parents and children and
by healthcare providers not supporting and even actively discouraging
women from breastfeeding.

At multiple levels (from individual to national), in multiple domains
(such as at home or locations where food is accessed or available), and
across multiple scales of time and space, there is a cumulative interplay
between exposure, susceptibility, and resistance (Krieger 2001, 2005; Yamada & Palmer 2006) to obesity among Choctaws. Factors include limited access to fresh produce; increased consumption of processed foods
high in fat, calories, and sugar; and lack of opportunities (accessibility,
availability, and time) for physical activity. Additionally, the associated
conditions of obesity—including hypertension, hyperlipidemia, hyper-
glycemia, and the increased risks associated with high waist-to-hip ratio
and cardiovascular disease, type 2 diabetes, and cerebrovascular disease—
also play a role in limiting physical activity. Plus, the high poverty and low
education rates combined with scarce or inappropriate work options prevent many tribal citizens from improving their socio-economic statuses,
which might otherwise allow them to purchase healthier foods. Finally,

the immune systems of Choctaws who experienced historical trauma and perceived threats (e.g., food scarcity, unemployment, monetary shortage, or illness) are adversely affected by psychosocial stressors, contributing to increased cortisol and visceral obesity (Wiley 1992).

The interplay between exposure, susceptibility, and resistance also involves the Choctaw Nation health services, including the availability and accessibility of relevant nutritional education. Run by the tribe, the health clinics and hospitals are staffed primarily by physicians participating in loan repayment programs and/or foreign-trained physicians who need work visas, many of whom lack cultural competence, cultural humility, and/or understanding of the socio-cultural, historical, and political-economic factors specific to Choctaws. Widely circulating and easily available resources aimed at supporting diabetics (e.g., diabetes wellness centers, medical shoes and other devices, nutrition assistance, etc.) also play a pivotal role in articulating a diabetic identity for Choctaws and, arguably, may work to create the very conditions that they sought to improve in the first place. With land alienation—dispossession of land through forced removal, the transference or change of ownership, title, or the denial of access to allotted Choctaw lands—Choctaws have experienced loss of traditional subsistence lifestyles, dependency on commodity foods, and even changes in food tastes and preferences. Land alienation is also directly related to decreased physical activity, as people no longer work outdoors, tend to crops or animals, or grow their own foods, for example, and it is therefore associated with an increased consumption of processed foods.

Embodied Heritage Framework

To examine the ways in which obesity is experienced, embodied, and made sense of within these multiple constraints on individual and collective agency, the embodied heritage framework brings together theoretical grounding and methods from Native American Indigenous Studies, critical biocultural and medical anthropology, historical trauma research, and heritage studies. Embodied heritage allows for an examination of how (or which) references of inequality, discrimination, and poverty today and/or in the past are selectively remembered; evoked; how they "get under the skin"; and how they dialectically shape collective memories, lived experiences, and understandings of individual and group identity.

Critical biocultural anthropology scholars have documented the ways in which political-economic inequalities and increasing wealth disparities contribute to negative health outcomes (Dressler 1993; Goodman et al. 1998; Gravlee et al. 2005; Leatherman 2005; Lock 2001; McDade 2002; Wiedman 2012), with much of the scholarship focusing on the ways in which stress from structural inequalities functions as a major contributor to poor health. These studies indeed document the ways in which inequality "gets under the skin," illuminating how larger structural factors figure into social processes and individual health. This project builds on work by these scholars, adding the perspective of meaning-making: the ways in which people make sense of these larger connections and the ways in which this meaning-making underpins identity and relationality. Specifically, embodied heritage focuses on meaning-making, personal and public narratives, and cultural identities, thus allowing for an examination of obesity at the intersections of issues related to structural, symbolic, and everyday violence, identity, heritage narratives, and historical trauma. It examines not whether obesity is more biological or more cultural, but "how these processes emerge and intersect as part of the biocultural dance" (Leatherman and Goodman 2011:30).

Understanding these social processes calls for understanding how local narratives explaining health inequities, such as obesity and diabetes (Ferreira and Lang 2006; Gittelsohn et al. 1996), often focus on the underlying role of historical trauma. Research links negative health effects of past traumatic events to subsequent generations (BraveHeart 1998, 1999; Evans-Campbell 2008) and, importantly, demonstrates that *how* people think about their personal histories and their collective pasts directly affects their health outcomes (Whitbeck et al. 2004). These studies underscore the value of narrative research to understand how (and which) representations of the past are evoked and used to explain health (Lang 2006; Mohatt et al. 2014).

This framework utilizes Smith's (2006:276) conceptualization of heritage as the "process of remembering that underpins identity and the ways in which individuals and groups make sense of their experiences in the present." Importantly, heritage is an active process (Dicks 2000; Graham et al. 2000; Lowenthal 1985; Smith 2006). It is an active process that is found in everyday life, including "just being together" and eating food together. This is a critical point, as this book examines not only what Choctaws identify as heritage, but why, how, and when this heritage-making occurs and, further, how it dialectally interacts with human biologies and health.

A note on identity: The term *identity* often suggests a fixed, individualistic notion of self, ignoring the intricate relationships that inform who we are and how we relate to ourselves and each other. In reality, identity is a dynamic process rooted in connections with family, community, land, and our environments and ecosystems. I prefer Kim TallBear's (2020) use of *relationality* when thinking through the loaded term *identity*. By centering the complexity of relationality in processes of identity-making, it allows for an acknowledgement of ongoing relating among individuals as part of a broader social and ecological network in ways that the term *identity* does not necessarily imply. Language choice is powerful, shaping and reflecting understandings and meanings. I hope to use the term *identity* with more precision and intent to ensure that the collective nature of Choctaw *relationality* is not obscured by narrower interpretations of *identity* as a mere individual trait or choice—the goal being to highlight *not* a strictly personal dimension of identity, but rather the nexus of our experiences, concerns, stories, and ways of knowing and being as situated in relationality. In other words, in what ways do memories, experiences, forms of violence, collective narratives, and foodways serve as conduits for identity-making and belonging (through kinship, collectivity, or other communal bonds) among Choctaws? It's about a collective narrative more than a solitary one; it's a focus not on the lens of personal identity, but rather on a deeper collective significance that includes relating with humans and non-humans as well (TallBear 2020).

An embodied heritage framework emphasizes that current experiences of obesity, diabetes, and related conditions are not isolated events disconnected in time from our collective past. They are part of a long process, the ongoing structure of settler-colonialism, and must include the perspective of meaning-making to understand how larger structural factors figure into social processes and individual health. Put simply, the concept of embodied heritage posits that health is contingent on one's social, economic, historical, cultural, and political position *and* the structures of meaning that make sense of this personal and embodied experience.

Commod Bod

"Commod bod," a term used to link large bodies with high-calorie, high-fat food commodities, is used humorously and is an example of in-group teasing about fat bodies. Across social media, there are a variety of "commod bod" cultural examples, including T-shirts and online forums for sharing pictures, stories, and memes about "commod bods." There is even a comic series: Super Indian, about a superhero who got his power from eating tainted government cheese, and his trusty sidekick Mega Bear, who is notorious for his "commod bod" (Starr 2012). Further, while the "commod bod" originates in relation to government-issued commodity foods, its usage has expanded to describe broader patterns of embodiment shaped by the consumption of calorie-dense, high-fat foods—whether or not they come from official commodity programs. For example, one woman I interviewed was eating a large roast beef sandwich from Arby's, the sauce running down her hand as we talked about foods, obesity, and identity. She laughed, pointed to the sandwich (even licked off the dripping sauce!) and commented that she was "working on her 'commod bod.'"

Notably, the term "commod bod" is used playfully and as a signifier for obesity, but it also does another kind of work: "Commod bod"—the term itself and the ways it is used—links present experiences of loss of food sovereignty, fat bodies, poverty, and disenfranchisement with the past by actively calling on specific material culture (i.e., commodity foods and "commod bods") produced in response to past injustices. It reflects the reality of shifting food sovereignty from self-sufficiency to lack of control over food systems; this links historical trauma with contemporary forms of violence. The use of this term alters inquiries surrounding large bodies away from medical and public health discourses to social and cultural discourses. Moreover, it serves as a marker for Indianness by linking commodities and poor food environments with large bodies. Darla,[13] a woman I interviewed during my exploratory fieldwork, shared this sentiment with me when describing a connectedness between obesity and Indianness: "When I'm around other Indians, the really traditional Indians, and we're all overweight, I feel like it's okay to be fat. I feel more Indian." She went on to describe how she felt a connection with other Natives from across dozens of different tribal nations because they shared a sense of relatedness through embodied colonialism—through the "commod bods" that are physical manifestations of a shared past and current contemporary violences.

The use of the term "commod bod" then, evokes a past in ways that acknowledge collective suffering while at the same time wrestling back a sense of control. "Commod bods" come from a shared Indian experience of land and livelihood disenfranchisement, but they are symbolic of resistance and accepted as part of the collective in particular ways. Through the use of the term, people are interacting with the past while staying rooted in the present (Loulanski 2006). They are creating heritage by attributing meaning and value and even selecting what is to become remembered (Smith 2006).

"Commod bods" indeed symbolize terrible fallout from government policies, but they also symbolize a kind of power and resilience, the taking back of meaning and value. Furthermore, they get at the embodiment of heritage—the lived experiences of heritage. This is what the embodied heritage framework aims to really get at: the heritage we don't often talk about; heritage in familiar, everyday contexts; and heritage that "gets under the skin"—embodied heritage. When we open up the possibility for talking about heritage as a process found in the familiar, then we can allow space for the daily practices that bind us together: the lived experiences of heritage, of identity-making, of relationality. "Commod bod" is one such heritage-making concept that considers larger historical, social, and political-economic factors to provide understandings of ways Choctaws create heritage. By understanding how Choctaws embody both colonial histories and cultural resilience, linking heritage and health in local contexts, makes space for us to situate health as an interaction with the past through the present, allowing then for a recalibration of our understandings about obesity among Choctaws and about Indigenous health more generally.

Overview of Chapters

The remainder of this book is organized as follows. Chapter 1 provides a brief history of Choctaw relocation to Oklahoma through which I describe the long-standing demographic, economic, and political presence of Choctaws in the state and region and position the project within the fabric of southeastern Oklahoma's cultural landscape. I discuss what makes the Choctaw Nation a unique region in the United States. I also introduce the women interviewed for this project, providing a brief sociodemographic sketch of my interlocutors, as they make up some of the poorest people living in the state (and country), relying on the Food Distribution Program on Indian Reservations as a primary food source for their households.

In chapter 2, I investigate how individuals use narrative to make sense of their lived experiences, and why narratives are useful tools for developing this embodied heritage framework. The intersections of historical trauma, structural violence, and heritage- and identity-making fundamental to an embodied heritage framework will be illustrated through two women's food-centered life stories. Linda, a diabetic, has faced profound personal and social suffering—including poverty, racism, alcoholism, and abandonment—while also serving as the primary caregiver for her grandson. Sherry is a retired data processor who now cares full-time for her ailing sister. Though active in her church and community, she quietly carries trauma and shame. Renowned for sewing traditional Choctaw dresses, her work offers unique insight into the changing sizes of Choctaw bodies. Both Linda and Sherry have depended on government-supplied foods for as long as they can recall. These food-centered life stories introduce the reader to the women in this study and are analyzed to demonstrate the key dimensions of an embodied heritage framework. In doing so, this chapter shows the interconnections of the many processes foundational to embodied heritage.

Chapter 3 focuses on historical trauma and the prevalence and role of this framework across Indigenous health issues. Scholars across disciplines have employed constructs of historical trauma to describe the impacts and legacies of colonization, cultural and material dispossession, and historical oppression among Natives. This chapter introduces the discourses surrounding historical trauma, as well as critiques of using that focus as an explanatory model for health outcomes, behaviors, and disease trends among Indigenous peoples. Second, I explore the food-centered life history narratives to illustrate how experiences of historical trauma figure into women's meaning-making and to understand the role of historical trauma in the reporting of the narrative themes that emerged from them. I then present and unpack Nelly Coyote's story around these themes. Finally, I contend that historical trauma, and specifically the ways it's made sense of (as public narrative), cannot be dissociated from contemporary forms of violence, and that together they are the root of poor health within this population.

Chapter 4 presents the major themes around the social processes of heritage and identity described in women's life stories, complemented with a deeper understanding of meaning-making, which is the heart of the embodied heritage framework and demonstrates how women's experiences figure into the connections between obesity and identity among Choctaws. The chapter begins with a brief overview of what Laurajane Smith (2006) has called the "authorized heritage discourse," which privileges expert values over those of community and local interests and which works to constrain understandings of heritage as primarily material. Then, I unpack the most prevalent experiences that women described in their food-centered life history narratives as related to Indianness (markers of identity) and notions of heritage. Based on analysis of their stories, I then demonstrate how meaning-making illuminates the ways in which larger structural factors figure into social processes and individual health, as well as how people make sense of these connections in the construction of cultural identity. This chapter shows how embodied heritage frames health as contingent on one's social, economic, historical, cultural, and political position *and* the structures of meaning that make sense of this personal and embodied experience.

In chapter 5, I bring together concepts of food, identity, and belonging found across women's food-centered life stories to examine the association of obesity and identity in the lives of Choctaw women. This chapter frames and discusses the ways that foods and foodways impact notions of obesity, identity, and belonging within the contexts of historical trauma; structural, symbolic, and everyday violence; and heritage narratives. I begin by presenting cultural and traditional foods and foodways as described by participants, followed by the ways they link these with obesity. Next, I examine the Food Distribution Program on Indian Reservations (FDPIR) at a local level and describe an everyday shopping experience at one FDPIR store, followed by women's accounts of their FDPIR experiences. Then, I offer women's understandings of obesity (and related conditions) and the ways they make sense of the linkages between obesity and Choctaw identity. Finally, I include findings from the Body Image Assessment Scale and the Native American Acculturation Scale, collected for this research, and interpret them alongside women's narratives to demonstrate how larger social forces figure into possible mechanisms linking obesity and identity. In doing so, I demonstrate which social forces are at the heart of the embodied heritage framework and discuss the broader implications of embodied heritage apart from obesity.

The final chapter presents a summary of the findings, which demonstrate that how people think about their personal and collective pasts directly affects their health outcomes. Adding to other studies that underscore the value of understanding how (and which) representations of the past are evoked and used to explain health (Blackstock et al. 2006; Ferreira and Lang 2006; Mohatt et al. 2014; Scheder 2006; Whitbeck et al. 2004), the findings summarized in this chapter come together to illustrate that Choctaws recall past traumatic events, both as public narrative and personal experiences, as a way to make sense of what they identify in the present: interrupted traditions and reimagined Choctaw culture expressed in the day-to-day. This finding is essential because it informs local narratives that explain health inequities, specifically obesity and related conditions. Rather than simply stating that obesity is a marker of Indianness, the women identified the trifecta of struggle, poverty, and discrimination as markers of Indianness, and they understood obesity as the physical outcome or the embodiment of those experiences. These are experiences which are marked by poor food environments and a continued dependence on government-supplied foods, as well as cultural and material dispossession (i.e., loss of land, language, traditions, cultural expressions, knowledge, and stories). Finally, I discuss the larger implications of an embodied heritage framework and conclude with acknowledgement of the current efforts the Choctaw Nation is undertaking around issues of food and health.

CHAPTER 1

Historicizing, Politicizing, and Situating Obesity in the Choctaw Nation

Though not our original ancestral homelands, Choctaws have been an integral part of Oklahoma's history since before statehood, despite repeated efforts to continuously uproot the Choctaw people. The strong cultural, economic, and political presence of Choctaws has indelibly shaped the region. Even the state's name, Oklahoma, is of Choctaw origin. In *Chahta anumpa* (the Choctaw language), *okla* translates to "people," and *humma* can mean "red," so the term *Oklahumma* is often translated to "Red People" (*Biskinik* 2010).[1] The name persists today, as do many other Choctaw words for places in southeastern Oklahoma, all named to reflect the landscape's unique characteristics, available resources, usage, and notable historical events—a poignant testament to Choctaw survivance and connection with this new environment.

Choctaws were the first Southeastern tribe forcibly removed from our original lands in what is present-day Mississippi and relocated to Indian Territory (Oklahoma). However, the U.S. government's aggressive policies of Choctaw land acquisition can be traced back to the early 1800s, even before the Indian Removal Act of 1830 under President Andrew Jackson's administration. The devastating journey of Removal, often referred to as the "Trail of Tears" or "Trail of Tears and Death," is a defining period in Choctaw history, and in commemoration, historical markers map the route of Removal.[2] These markers, some more visible than others,

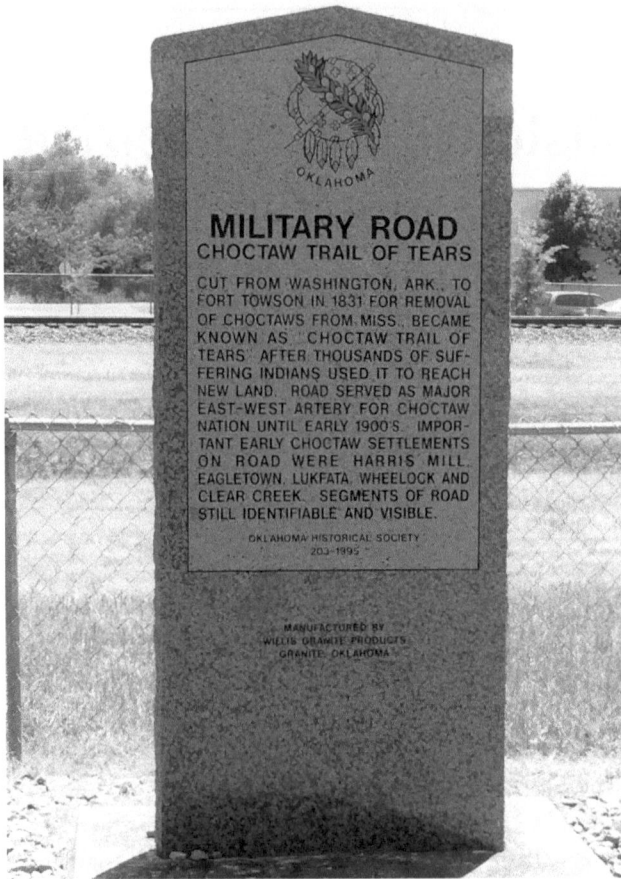

FIGURE 4 Military Road historical marker. Photo by Kasey Jernigan (author).

serve as poignant reminders of the multiple pathways, roads, and the "end" of the Trail that Choctaw people traversed during forced migration.

Oklahoma has the largest American Indian *alone* population (14 percent); the second largest population of American Indians *in combination* (16 percent); and the Choctaw Nation of Oklahoma has the third largest population of American Indians *alone* (3 percent) of all the federally recognized Indigenous nations (U.S. Census Bureau 2020).[3] Oklahoma has one of the most complex and significant tribal jurisdictional landscapes in the United States. This stems from its history as Indian Territory,

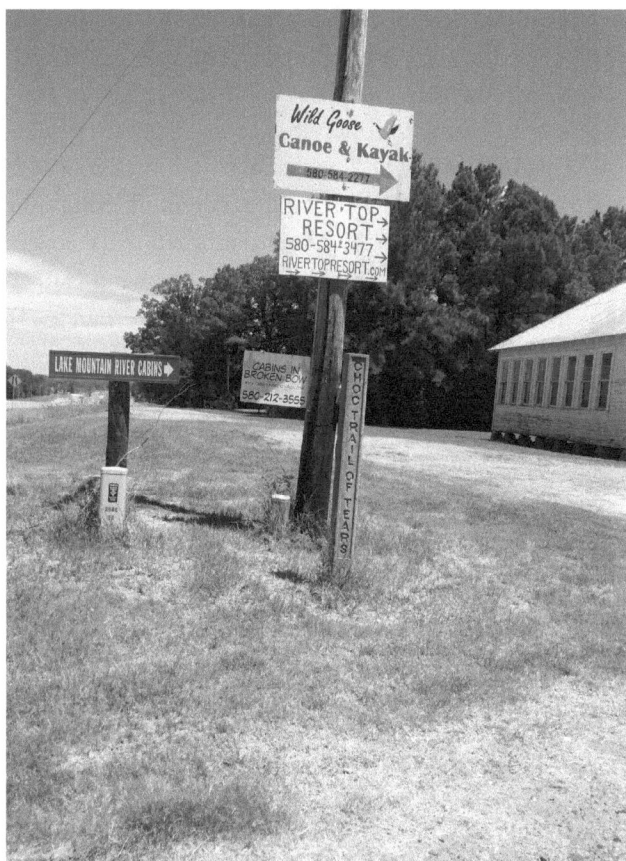

FIGURE 5 Trail of Tears historical marker, located under a sign giving directions to the River Top Resort. Photo by Kasey Jernigan (author).

where numerous tribes were forcibly relocated, and the legal precedents set by treaties, federal policies, and recent court rulings. Recognized as domestic dependent nations, the Supreme Court ruled in July 2020 in the case of *McGirt v. Oklahoma* that the eastern half of Oklahoma remains an Indian reservation for jurisdictional purposes (Healy and Liptak 2020; Rubin 2020).[4] This area encompasses the lands of the Chickasaw, Choctaw, Cherokee, Muscogee, and Seminole Nations, and the tribes govern their respective historical reservations, even though much of the land is now privately owned. The ruling was based on an 1832 treaty, which the court determined is still valid, stating, "Because Congress has not said otherwise, we hold the government to its word" (*McGirt v. Oklahoma* 2020). Consequently, the Choctaw Nation's status has reverted from that of a tribal jurisdictional area to a legally recognized Indian reservation.[5] The *McGirt v. Oklahoma* ruling—while primarily applicable to the Muscogee Creek Nation—set a precedent affecting other tribes, including the Choctaw Nation, and has reinforced tribal sovereignty by affirming tribal jurisdiction over major crimes involving Native citizens, challenging state authority, and expanding self-governance. The ruling has strengthened tribes' abilities to govern their own lands, enforce their laws, and shape their futures without external interference. However, as Roberts (2021, 2023) and Waldman (2023) emphasize, this sovereignty has also been selectively applied in ways that reinforce racial hierarchies.

The Five Tribes—Choctaw, Cherokee, Chickasaw, Creek, and Seminole—were among the Indigenous nations that enslaved people of African descent before the Civil War. Following Emancipation, the 1866 Reconstruction Treaties between these tribes and the U.S. government granted Freedmen citizenship within their respective nations (Littlefield 1978; Roberts 2023; Saunt 2004; Thomas 2024). However, over time, these rights were eroded through legal and political maneuvers, as tribal governments sought to reassert control over their membership criteria (Roberts 2021; Saunt 2004; Thomas 2024). In the Choctaw Nation, Freedmen and their descendants were initially recognized as tribal citizens after the 1866 treaty, but in 1983 they were stripped of their status, along with access to tribal resources, healthcare, land allotments, and political participation (Herrera 2021). This exclusion has persisted— descendants of Choctaw Freedmen without documented lineage to a Choctaw individual listed on the final Dawes Rolls are denied tribal citizenship—even as the Choctaw Nation has expanded its economic and political influence. While the Cherokee Nation restored Freedmen citizenship rights in 2017, the Choctaw, Chickasaw, Creek, and Seminole Nations continue to deny full membership to Freedmen descendants, arguing that tribal sovereignty gives them the authority to define their own citizenry (Roberts 2023).[6]

The population within the geographical boundaries of the Choctaw Nation—the region included in this project—is approximately 26 percent Native (U.S. Census Bureau 2020). This population, although majority Choctaw, is not static and includes a mixture of tribes and non-Native peoples from different regions, cultures, educational backgrounds, and stories of assimilation. According to the 2020 Census, more than 20 percent of this population lives below the poverty line—compared with 15 percent in the state of Oklahoma and 12 percent in the United States—with some counties reporting a greater than 50 percent poverty rate (U.S. Census 2020). The women interviewed for this project depend on food from the Food Distribution locations spread across the reservation—food which is intended to be supplementary (Story et al. 1999) rather than a primary food source (Dillinger 1999). This study depicts women's experiences within the southeastern Oklahoma Native population that struggles at or below the poverty line. However, it specifically examines the experiences of impoverished Choctaws in the region and does not claim to reflect Oklahoma Natives at large.

In this chapter, I discuss what makes the Choctaw reservation a unique region in the United States, including the current demographic and economic contributions of the Choctaw Nation, and provide a brief history of Choctaw removal, relocation, and assimilation. Then I describe the project setting and population of women interviewed. Finally, I provide a brief sociodemographic sketch of the women who shared their stories with me.

Demographic and Economic Data

The Choctaw Nation of Oklahoma is the largest of the three federally recognized bands of Choctaws, with more than 225,000 enrolled citizens, of which approximately 85,000 live in the state of Oklahoma (OK Indian Affairs Commission 2011). In other words, more than three-quarters of Oklahoma Choctaws reside outside of the Choctaw Nation Reservation and the state of Oklahoma. The reasons for such widespread dispersal vary, with families having their own narratives of voluntary or involuntary migration, yet relocation to urban centers is a common theme (*Biskinik* 2024) that is important to the heritage component of the embodied heritage framework and will be described later in this chapter.

The Choctaw reservation is defined as an extremely rural, ten-and-a-half-county territory spanning almost eleven thousand square miles

FIGURE 6 Map of Oklahoma. The Choctaw Nation is highlighted in the southeastern part of the state. Courtesy of Wikimedia Commons User Tcr25 | CC BY-SA 4.0 https://creativecommons.org/licenses/by-sa/4.0/.

(U.S. Census Bureau 2020) in southeastern Oklahoma, which encompasses about 15 percent of the state's total area. The reservation includes mountains, rivers, lakes, and woodlands with ample fishing, hunting, and natural resources. The Choctaw Nation's service area includes the ten-and-a-half counties, the second largest tribal service area in the lower forty-eight states (U.S. Census Bureau 2011).[7] To put the vastness of the reservation into perspective, it is larger than seven U.S. states, and it takes about three hours (160 miles) to travel from the southwest to the northeast corner of the reservation.[8] Not only is the territory vast, but southeast Oklahoma is a largely rural region that is more mountainous and forested than any other part of the state (CNO Economic and Demographic Data 2016).

According to the CNO, the Choctaw service area is home to approximately 53,000 Native Americans, accounting for as much as 50 percent of the population in some communities, about 42,000 (approximately 80 percent) of whom are reported as Choctaw by the Tribal Membership Office (CNO Economic and Demographic Data 2016). The remaining Native population in this area is made up of as many as twenty-nine different tribes, making this a diverse region with many languages, dialects, and cultures.[9]

In 2014, the Choctaw Nation was designated as the first Tribal *Promise Zone* under the Obama Administration (Hall 2015). This designation highlights the region's significant challenges, including extreme poverty, high levels of unemployment, and low educational attainment. Southeastern Oklahoma has some of the poorest counties in both the state and the country. All ten-and-a-half counties within the Choctaw Nation have also been identified as USDA StrikeForce Areas (USDA 2015), a federal program which targets the most economically distressed regions in the country to assist in economic development (USDA Strikeforce Initiative 2015; CNO 2016).

LeFlore, Latimer, and McCurtain counties within the Choctaw Nation rank first, second, and third, respectively, for the highest unemployment rates in the state, and these counties also have the largest Native American populations (Oklahoma Employment Security Commission 2015). However, unemployment rates alone do not fully capture the severity of the region's economic hardships. Workers in southeastern Oklahoma are among the lowest paid in the state, with average annual salaries significantly below both the state and national averages (CNO Economic and Demographic Data 2016). Those who are employed often hold minimum wage jobs, with the average weekly wage in the region being 32 percent lower than the national average (U.S. Census Bureau 2020).

Historian Arlen M. Hanson (2021:277) explains that before forced removal, Choctaws engaged in diverse economic activities not merely as acts of acculturation but as deliberate strategies to sustain sovereignty. As some of the largest cotton producers and cattle ranchers in Mississippi, they invested in industrial development (such as blacksmith shops) for economic gain, to reduce dependence on American goods, and as a way to achieve self-sufficiency. An often-overlooked reality of this was Choctaw reliance on enslaved African Americans. As Alaina E. Roberts (2021) details, Choctaw elites were among the largest slaveholders in the southeastern U.S. before removal, with enslaved laborers working on Choctaw-owned plantations, producing cotton, and maintaining livestock. This economic entanglement did not end with removal; when the Choctaw were forcibly relocated to Indian Territory, many of these enslaved individuals remained under Choctaw ownership, complicating traditional narratives of aggressive United States–Indigenous relations

(Roberts 2023). While the Choctaw Council's vision of economic self-sufficiency as a means of preserving sovereignty was disrupted by removal, it was not abandoned. Nearly two centuries later, the Choctaw Nation in Oklahoma continues to pursue diversified economic enterprises to sustain its sovereignty, carrying forward the ambitions of its pre-removal leaders. Yet, this ongoing economic success remains tied to a complex history in which sovereignty and self-sufficiency were built on systems of oppression.[10]

The Choctaw Nation is decidedly a major economic driver in the region and state. In 2021, its annual tribal economic impact was $3.2 billion, and the tribe is the largest employer in southeastern Oklahoma, with more than 12,000 employees and 20,142 jobs supported (CNO Economic Development Partnership 2021). The Nation manages a diverse range of businesses, including eight casinos, fourteen tribal smoke shops, thirteen travel plazas (gas stations/truck stops), two Chili's restaurants located in Atoka and Poteau, and Reba's Place, a dining and entertainment venue constructed in partnership with country singer Reba McEntire.[11] Additionally, the Nation operates a variety of enterprises such as a printing company, a corporate drug testing service, hospice care and senior living developments, a metal fabrication and manufacturing business, a document backup and archival service, and a management services firm that provides staffing for military bases, embassies, and other locations.

The largest single business operation is the Choctaw Casino and Resort Sky Tower ("the Resort Casino"), the flagship of the Nation's gaming industry, located in Durant. The $860 million Resort Casino employs nearly 2,500 people and hosts over three million visitors per year, two-thirds of whom originate from the Dallas–Fort Worth metroplex.[12] Tourism spending over the last five years has increased by 64 percent in the CNO, with annual travel spending reaching $1.8 billion in 2021 (CNO Economic Development Partnership Annual Report 2022). Tourists visit for the casinos but also for camping, wineries, state parks, scenic drives, music festivals, cultural events, rodeos, museums, and more, with the CNO leading the state in tourism growth (CNO Economic Development Partnership Annual Report 2022).

Business revenues from these businesses are invested in tribal government and community services, including Choctaw Transportation, the Choctaw Day Care and Head Start Center, and the Food Distribution

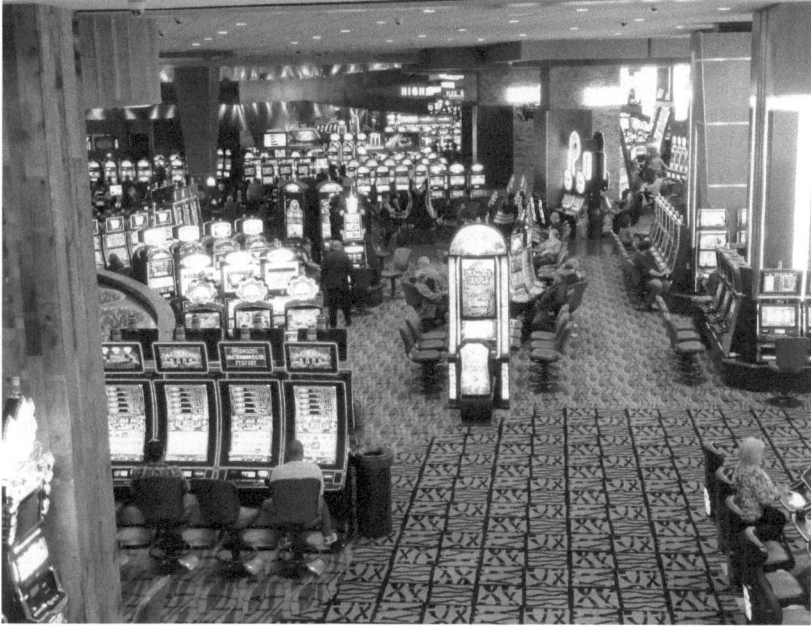

FIGURE 7 Slot machines inside the Resort Casino, Durant, Oklahoma. Photo by Kasey Jernigan (author).

stores. According to Dara McCoy, Grants Director at CNO, "business revenue generated is reinvested by the Choctaw Nation throughout the tribal service area to improve the quality of life and battle immense socio-economic challenges throughout the federally designated Promise Zone. Programs funded by this revenue include higher education scholarships, college and career training, certification and preparatory services, student services, victims of crime advocacy and services, vocational rehabilitation, youth empowerment and intervention programs, children and family services, maternal and infant home visits, Head Start and Early Head Start, and many more life-changing services" (personal communication April 3, 2016).

Tribal revenue is also invested locally to build water systems and towers, roads, and other infrastructure and has contributed to additional fire stations, EMS units, and law enforcement needs that have accompanied this fast economic growth. The Choctaw Nation's economic impact on the state is profound: In 2021 alone, the Nation supported more than

20,000 Oklahoma jobs, with over $1 billion in wages and benefits paid to Oklahomans; contributed more than $3.5 million to cities and counties across the state; invested $11.1 million in Oklahoma highways and roads; invested $61 million in education funding; paid $335 million in exclusivity fees since 2005,[13] with $34.2 million to support education in 2021; paid $282 million in health spending; and recycled more than four million pounds of waste. In other words, the Choctaw Nation, along with other tribes in the state, are substantial economic drivers in Oklahoma, the bedrocks of commerce in many rural communities. They help to stabilize local economies and contribute to local and state needs such as schools and infrastructure.

Though beyond the scope of this project, there is much to unpack around the ways that economic development through gaming and other business endeavors can serve as both a tool for empowerment and a site of negotiation for Choctaw sovereignty. Gaming and participation in global capitalism—the revenue from these endeavors, to be exact—has made possible Choctaw financial independence, strengthened Choctaw political power, and allowed for resistance to federal and state encroachments on Choctaw sovereignty.[14] As anthropologist Jessica Cattelino's (2010) work with the Seminole Nation highlights, gaming has not only been a tool for economic uplift but also a significant cultural and political strategy that challenges traditional notions of sovereignty and self-determination in Indigenous communities. As with the Seminole Nation, there is a complex interplay between economic practices and cultural identity in the Choctaw Nation, showing how tribes with economic self-sufficiency navigate and negotiate their autonomy within the broader context of U.S. federalism.

McAlester has historically been the largest city within the Nation, serving as its main business hub. However, by the 2020 U.S. Census, Durant had surpassed McAlester in population, largely due to the Nation's governmental headquarters being located there. Opened in June 2018, the new headquarters replaced the previous, which was housed in the former Oklahoma Presbyterian College and included several key offices scattered around Durant. The new headquarters is an impressive five-story, 500,000 square foot building located on an eighty-acre campus in south Durant. The complex includes the Tribal Member Services and government headquarters and provides a "one-stop" resource for tribal members for medical services, prescriptions, tribal membership information, and scholarship and employment training programs. It is situated near other tribal buildings, such as the regional health clinic, wellness center, community center, child development center, and Food Distribution store.

Historical Context

Essentially the "test case" for Indian removal, the Choctaws of the Southeast were the first to be removed under the Indian Removal Act of 1830. Now commonly referred to as the "Trail of Tears" or "Trail of Tears and Death," this forced migration had devastating impacts on the tribes involved. Removal covered approximately five hundred miles and took place in three main waves (1831–1833), though there were many more smaller removals throughout the nineteenth century, rendering Choctaw removal a decades-long reality (Hanson 2021; Roberts 1986). Poor planning, inadequate supplies and funding, and harsh winter weather led to perilous conditions and resulted in cholera, starvation, and death, decimating the tribe. Estimates report around 15,000 Choctaws were removed from the Southeast, with death toll estimates ranging from 2,500–6,000 (Akers 2004; DeRosier 1970; Foreman 1932; Schultz et al. 2016).[15]

Upon resettlement in Indian Territory (present-day Oklahoma), Choctaws occupied small parcels of land within the original 6.8-million-acre tribal estate granted through the Treaty of Dancing Rabbit Creek and subsisted mainly through small-scale farming, animal husbandry, hunting, and fishing (Faiman-Silva 1993, 2000; Lambert 2007). However, by the early 1950s, Choctaw land ownership had dwindled to just about eleven thousand acres, mostly in scattered tracts of about twenty acres or less (Debo 1972; Faiman-Silva 1993, 2000), a consequence of both federal allotment policies and the encroachment of non-Native settlers.

Initially, the Five Civilized Tribes, including the Choctaws, were exempt from the Dawes Act of 1887, which aimed to break up tribal lands and assimilate Natives into the U.S. private property system. The exemption was because the Five Tribes had negotiated treaties with the U.S. government that recognized their land as communal and sovereign.

Tribes controlled their land collectively under the terms of their treaties with the U.S. and continued to maintain their own governments,
legal systems, and land tenure structures in Indian Territory. However,
pressure from the federal government and non-Native settlers seeking
access to land in Indian Territory led to the passage of the Curtis Act
of 1898, which directly targeted the Five Tribes, abolished their tribal
courts and legal systems, and forcibly applied the allotment process to
their lands. With the Curtis Act's forced allotment, the Choctaw Nation
lost millions of acres, as land was redistributed into private allotments for
enrolled members, reinforcing a system that privileged certain individuals while disadvantaging others.[16] Even before formal allotment, white
settlers illegally fenced off and claimed Choctaw land in direct violation
of existing treaties, and by the 1907 Five Tribes census, Choctaws were
vastly outnumbered by white settlers (9 percent compared to 79 percent), many of whom had entered the Nation illegally (Faiman-Silva 1993,
2000). The passage of the 1908 Restrictions Act then facilitated the sale
of over half of the Choctaw Nation's original estate to outsiders, acceler-
ating land dispossession (Debo 1972; Faiman-Silva 1993). This transformation mirrored broader shifts in rural America: As small-scale farming
declined between 1929 and 1959—dropping by more than 50 percent
in McCurtain County and over 60 percent in Pushmataha County—
land ownership became increasingly concentrated in private hands and
timber companies, while Choctaws entered the cash economy through
government-subsidized employment, Works Projects Administration
jobs, and military service (Faiman-Silva 1993). Faiman-Silva (pp. 47–48)
notes, "As it had been since the allotment system's inception in 1902, land
was bargained in exchange for subsistence commodities, when necessary,
a practice that saw nearly complete Choctaw Nation land alienation by
1950." Without land for subsistence, there was a radical shift from agricultural self-sufficiency to reliance on wage labor and government food
commodities, which vastly altered Choctaw foodways and economic
independence.

Settler contact and relocation to Indian Territory brought a profound
change to Choctaw life, transforming the Nation from one formally
organized around kinship, interconnected and balanced roles, mixed
subsistence, and inter-tribal trade to one characterized by marked differences in wealth, market-oriented production, centralized leadership,

land loss, and citizenship (Faiman-Silva 1993; Lambert 2007; Moore 1993). According to Stephen Cornell (1988:56–62), the settlers had three hegemonic agendas in their encounters with Southeastern Indigenous peoples: to expropriate resources, to transform the culture through "civilization," and to gain political control by dismantling the nations. These were accomplished by various means in the Choctaw Nation—programs and policies whose aim was to integrate Choctaws into "Euro-American" values, norms, and practices were propelled by two "change agents"— missions and schools. Euro-American missionaries (mostly Presbyterian and Congregational, but some Methodist and Baptist) accompanied Choctaws during Removal and helped establish the first mission stations, which included educational and religious buildings and residential dwellings (Cornell 1988). The goal of the missions was to "teach common school learning and the useful arts of life and Christianity; [and] so gradually to make the whole tribe English in language, civilized in habits, and Christian in religion" (Morrison 1997:23). Mission-sponsored boarding schools were also constructed as yet another technique to assimilate Choctaws. Many graduates of these boarding schools went on to participate in the government-sponsored urban relocation programs of the 1940s–1960s, further contributing to the depopulation of the CNO (Faiman-Silva 1997). Ultimately, the tribe became a "domestic dependent nation . . . completely under the sovereignty and dominion of the U.S." (Faiman-Silva 1997:6), struggling to retain legitimate national sovereignty and cultural integrity, while the U.S. government continued its own agenda of separating Choctaws from the land and assimilating them into mainstream society.

Indian Health, Choctaw Health: Federal Indian Trust Responsibility and Assimilation Policies

Native Americans have unique legal rights to federal health care services, a legal relationship between tribes and the federal government that dates back to the eighteenth century, and which has significantly influenced the conditions that affect Indigenous health and well-being today. This relationship, rooted in a complex legal and constitutional framework, is understood as the federal Indian trust responsibility (Baciu et al. 2017;

Cohen 1982, U.S. Commission on Civil Rights 2004). As tribes ceded lands, the government assumed this responsibility, ratified in treaties, statutes, and court decisions, requiring the federal government to protect tribal lands, resources, and sovereignty (Calabrese 2024; Cohen 1982).[17] The trust doctrine was solidified in key cases, such as *Cherokee Nation v. Georgia* (1831), where tribes were described as "domestic dependent nations" under the care of the federal government. This fiduciary obligation extends to ensuring tribes' welfare, including the provision of essential services like healthcare (Baciu et al. 2017; Cohen 1982).

There is sparse evidence about Indian health problems prior to European contact, so much of what we do know comes from catastrophic outbreaks like smallpox, measles, influenza, and malaria and early colonial efforts to document these diseases (while providing opportunities to theorize why mortality was so high among Indians). David S. Jones, a physician and historian of medicine, writes that "estimates of pre-contact American populations vary between 8 and 112 million (two to twelve million for North America), and estimates of total mortality range from 7 to 100 million. Whatever the exact numbers, the mortality was unprecedented and overwhelming" (Jones 2006:2123). During the first century after contact, populations often decreased by more than 90 percent. As Mark Trahant writes, "It's impossible to overstate the consequences of a 90 percent mortality rate. This is the root of historical trauma: the collective memory of a people nearly wiped off of their homeland" (Trahant 2018:2–3).

Though largely speculative, estimates of the pre-contact and early contact Choctaw population range from 30,000 to 100,000. Between 1519 and 1672, at least seventeen pandemics, including smallpox, measles, typhus, plague, yellow fever, and influenza, devastated Indian communities in the Southeast (Smith 1992; Wang et al. 2004), causing significant population declines. In 1685, the Choctaw population was estimated at 28,000 (Wood 2006), but smallpox, warfare, and the slave trade had reduced their numbers to less than half that in just forty-five years (Wood 2006). The first U.S. census of the Choctaw in 1830, known as the Armstrong Roll and conducted before forced relocation to Indian Territory, recorded 19,544 individuals. By 1843, only 12,690 Choctaws were documented in Indian Territory. These are just numbers though, and they do not and cannot account for the Choctaws never born because of the genocide of these ancestors; nor for the loss of much cultural knowledge that died with Elders and other knowledge holders; and more, the ways that mass death, removal, loss, and assimilation affect Choctaw ways of knowing and being on their new land, for generations, rendering "social and cultural systems almost inoperative" (Akers 2004:94).

As tribes resettled on reservations, they continued to suffer from infectious diseases. In the 1900s, nascent federal efforts to provide healthcare programs on Native American reservations were largely ineffective and failed to address the critical health needs of tribal communities (US Commission on Civil Rights 2004). Underfunded and poorly managed, these programs did little to improve the dire health and sanitary conditions on reservations. Across tribes, communities continued to suffer from preventable and treatable diseases and lacked access to adequate medical services. These shortcomings led to the passage of the Snyder Act in 1921, which formally authorized federal healthcare for tribes but still faced implementation challenges (Shelton 2004). In 1955, the Indian Health Service (IHS) was established to fulfil the federal trust obligation of providing healthcare to Natives. It struggled with limited resources and infrastructure during this period, reflecting broader systemic neglect by the federal government (U.S. Commission on Civil Rights 2004).

Chronic underfunding and limited resources in federal programs like Indian Health Services continue to leave many tribal members without timely and adequate care, motivating the Choctaw Nation to take control of its nation's healthcare needs. With the many shortcomings of federal healthcare services available, the Choctaw Nation compacted with the federal government to provide healthcare services directly to Indians within its jurisdiction. In 1999, the Nation was the first tribe in the United States to build its own hospital, with its own funding (CNHSA 2016). The $22 million hospital, located in Talihina, is a 145,000-square-foot health facility with thirty-seven hospital beds and fifty-two exam rooms, which serves approximately 200,000 outpatient visits annually (CNHSA 2016). The hospital also houses the Choctaw Nation Health Services Authority (CNHSA), the hub of the tribal health care services of southeastern Oklahoma (CNHSA 2016). The Nation also operates eight outlying clinics across the reservation, in Atoka, Broken Bow, Durant, Hugo, Idabel, McAlester, Poteau, and Stigler. By building its own hospital, the Choctaw Nation aimed to provide high-quality, culturally sensitive healthcare that better serves the community's needs, emphasizing sovereignty and self-determination in addressing healthcare disparities (Shelton 2004). This decision reflects a broader trend among Native nations of assuming greater responsibility over their services and resources (NCAI 2020).

Assimilation policies of the late nineteenth century have had sustained effects on Indian communities and, ultimately, Indigenous health conditions (Baciu et al. 2017). Following early assimilation policies such as the General Allotment Act of 1887 and the Indian Boarding Schools systems—which banned cultural practices such as religions, healing methods, languages, dress, and hairstyles—U.S. federal policies toward tribal nations shifted toward reorganization. The U.S. government recognized that its efforts to assimilate Native peoples into mainstream American society had not been successful. The Indian Reorganization Act of 1934 (IRA) marked a significant change, aiming to promote economic development, self-governance, and modernized business practices within tribes (Shelton 2004). However, this period of tribal empowerment was relatively short-lived. By the 1950s, Congress was enacting legislation aimed at terminating its relationship with tribal nations through a policy known as Indian Termination. This policy sought to dismantle the special federal-tribal relationships, end recognition of tribal governments, withdraw government support for tribal nations, and eliminate the protected status of Indian-owned lands (Wilkins and Stark 2017). During this era, Congress enacted legislation that terminated the recognition of 109 tribes, removing their federal status and leading to the elimination of their reservations. The Choctaw Nation faced federal termination between 1959 and 1970, as the federal government began to withdraw support for essential services such as healthcare, education, utilities, and public safety and planned to sell off Choctaw assets through public auction. Grassroots activism in the 1970s reversed Termination (Lambert 2007), but this era had long-lasting consequences on tribal communities, particularly in areas such as mental health, cultural identity, and social networks, as tribal citizens were relocated to urban areas away from their tribal lands (Shelton 2004; Walls and Whitbeck 2012).

In 1956, Congress passed the Indian Relocation Act, legislation aimed at providing vocational training programs for Native Americans, which necessitated relocating people from their reservations to large urban centers. The Bureau of Indian Affairs initiated the Indian Urban Relocation

Program to facilitate this process, relocating Native families to major cities including Cleveland, Dallas, Los Angeles, Minneapolis, San Francisco, San Jose, and Seattle. Between 1950 and 1968, over 200,000 Native people were relocated under this program. Before 1956, only 6 percent of Native Americans lived in large cities, but by 2000, that figure had risen to over 64 percent (National Archives 2024). The Indian Urban Relocation Program promised various forms of assistance, including housing, employment, transportation, vocational training, and other incentives. However, in practice, these promises were often unfulfilled or discontinued once families had relocated, leading to widespread issues such as unemployment, low-wage jobs, discrimination, homesickness, homelessness, and a loss of cultural support systems. Specific to Choctaws, families and individuals were relocated to urban locations such as Oklahoma City, Tulsa, and Denver, but also as far away as Bakersfield, Calif., and Chicago (Burt 1986; Ramirez 2007; Snipp 1992).

Despite the immediate and long-term negative impacts such as isolation from home communities and increased segregation and discrimination (Garrett and Pichette 2000), relocatees in urban areas began forming inclusive communities that transcended tribal lines. These urban Indian communities emphasized shared experiences of displacement and developed a pan-Indian movement centered around unity and cultural revival. Urban Indian centers, social gatherings, and intertribal activities like powwows became key spaces for fostering a broader Indian identity grounded in solidarity and collective pride. The relocation also sparked political movements such as the American Indian Movement (AIM), which aimed to address shared issues like poverty, discrimination, and the fight for treaty rights and sovereignty. Today, more than 70 percent of Natives in the United States live in urban areas, with significant populations in Los Angeles, New York, Phoenix, and Anchorage. These experiences have given shape to a collective urban Indian identity—a complex identity which is related to disconnection from tribal lands and the need to navigate life in a predominantly non-Native environment while maintaining cultural ties and a sense of belonging to one's tribal affiliation *and* adapting to new and diverse tribal cultures and traditions.

Embodied experiences for Indigenous peoples are not contained within an individual body but within a social one that is defined and informed by relatedness and its practices (Heil 2008). As described in the Introduction, commodity food experiences (and "commod bods") are more than merely a shared experience among urban Indians. Commodity food experiences and the health conditions that come from these foods serve as an important way to overcome differences between tribal cultures while emphasizing similarities (Vantrese 2013). This dual process of overcoming differences and emphasizing similarities is foundational to an urban Indian identity, which gets asserted at diverse urban gatherings and everyday situations. In these experiences, people relate to each other: They are participating socially, the essence of a fundamentally interdependent personhood and the essence of what it means to be socially valued, Indigenous, and therefore well (Heil 2008).

Although the Choctaw Nation is a rural area, the reservation is populated with people from diverse tribes, and many Choctaws who live there have left for cities and returned with urban experiences. In these ways, the processes of overcoming differences and emphasizing similarities resonate for Choctaws in southeastern Oklahoma. We see this in the high rates of obesity and diabetes among Natives in the region (and across the United States in general) which, from a non-Indigenous perspective, does not necessarily point to a healthy or well individual (nor is it something that necessarily benefits the individual as an embodied self). But practices of health and wellness among Choctaws are ultimately sanctioned by the degree to which individuals are able to better locate the embodied self within the nexus of social relatedness (Burkitt 1991; Heil 2008). Fat or diabetic bodies serve as connector to other Indians, calling upon shared trauma and violences unique to Indians, across time and space.

The Choctaw Nation is still grappling with the repercussions of relocation and is working intentionally to mend the damages caused. The nation's leadership is now making strides to reconnect with its members, especially those who live outside the boundaries of the nation, by establishing various cultural programs and gatherings in cities across the United States, aimed at fostering these connections. A profound focus of these endeavors is the re-education of Choctaw people about history, stories, cultural ways, and the preservation of *Chahta anumpa*. Cultural ambassador Ryan Spring states, "The Choctaw Nation is rebuilding its relationship with the land and re-educating its members who lost their history, including their language. Deep wounds left by the removals of the Choctaw people are beginning to heal" (Plummer 2020). These efforts mark a significant step toward healing and restoration, providing hope for a future that fosters and celebrates the remembering and re-storying of Choctaw culture. As Heil (2008) argues, to experience wellness, showing up and "participating in the social are prerequisites" for Indigenous people. Therefore, showing up and participating in the social around remembering, (re)storying, and reclaiming Choctaw culture instead of connecting around trauma and violence should also affect the foci of relatedness and its practices.

Throughout the remainder of this book, I will return to this historical context and to settler colonialism as an ongoing structure (rather than a past historical event), which serves as the basis for a historically grounded and inclusive analysis of the various ways in which the development of a white settler U.S. state and political economy shaped Indigenous and Choctaw practices of relatedness, as well as health inequities (including obesity and related conditions) among Choctaws and Indians in general. I explore women's narratives of obesity that are intimately interconnected with structural violence, practices of relatedness, historical trauma and heritage, and meaning-making. By focusing on these stories, I hope to explain the ways shifting patterns of participation in food and nutrition assistance programs have shaped Choctaw foodways; how these foodways are linked to Choctaw bodies and health, particularly obesity and related conditions; and how foodways and bodies are intertwined with meaning-making of historical trauma and contemporary violence, identity, and heritage.

A Note on Methods

I used three forms of data collection during a seven-month period of fieldwork in 2016: mixed-method interviews and surveys involving semi-structured food-centered life history narratives; participant observation; and archival research. During interviews, women were asked about their behaviors, experiences, beliefs, and memories centered on food production, preservation, preparation, consumption, distribution, and exchange. I included prompts on, for example, past and present diets; recipes; everyday and ritual meals; foods for health and wellbeing; food memories;

TABLE 1 Socio-demographics of the sample population

Socio-Demographic Characteristics	Sample Population
Sample Size	49
Age Mean ± SD (in years) [Range]	51.7 ± 15.4 [18–70]
Blood Quantum Mean (% NA) [Range]*	51% ± 0.4 [1%–100%]
Tribal Heritages	
Choctaw only	42 (86%)
Choctaw + 1 other tribe	2 (4%)
Choctaw + 2 other tribes	1 (2%)
Other tribe(s)	4 (8%)
Marital Status	
Married	23 (47%)
Living with a partner	4 (8%)
Divorced	7 (14%)
Separated	1 (2%)
Widowed	7 (14%)
Never married	7 (14%)
Work Status	
Working full-time	23 (47%)
Working part-time	3 (6%)
Unemployed or laid off	4 (8%)
Does not work due to health reasons/disabled	5 (10%)
Retired	9 (18%)
Homemaker or raising children	1 (2%)
Student	2 (4%)
Other (caregiver)	2 (4%)
	(*continued*)

and processed versus fresh foods. I began each narrative interview with what I thought was a simple question: "Can you tell me what you ate yesterday from when you woke up to when you went to sleep?" Based on this question, and sometimes with more targeted probing such as "How did you prepare/obtain that food?" and "Can you describe where, when, and with whom you ate this?" many women launched into detailed descriptions of their food practices, family meals, and memories of food experiences growing up.[18] I also asked participants to complete six surveys to document variations across general health and well-being, the food and nutrition environment, acculturation, historical losses, body image, and socio-demographics.[19] I also measured the women's heights,

TABLE 1 (*continued*)

Socio-Demographic Characteristics	Sample Population
Level of Education	
No formal schooling	1 (2%)
Less than high school diploma or equivalency/GED	0 (0%)
High school diploma or equivalency/GED	18 (37%)
Some college or some technical college	16 (33%)
Associate's degree or technical college degree	6 (12%)
Four-year college, bachelor's degree, or higher	8 (16%)
Household Income	
Under $5,000	1 (2%)
$5,000–$9,999	3 (6%)
$10,000–$14,999	7 (14%)
$15,000–$19,999	5 (10%)
$20,000–$29,999	7 (14%)
$30,000–$39,999	7 (14%)
$40,000–$49,999	4 (8%)
$50,000–$59,000	2 (4%)
$60,000–$69,999	2 (4%)
$70,000–$79,999	1 (2%)
$80,000 or above	4 (8%)
Don't know or don't want to answer	6 (12%)

weights, and waist circumferences. While women's food-centered life stories are the focus of this book, these quantitative and anthropometric data provided rich insight into the relationships between obesity; the historical traumas/violences reported in their food-centered life history narratives; and more objective measures of health, obesity, and identity that are presented elsewhere (Jernigan 2018).

A general protocol was followed in which participants were recruited from the Food Distribution stores on five sites and given the option to participate in a one to three-hour interview in a private room at the store.[20] Very few eligible women declined to participate in the interview.[21] In some cases, women preferred to conduct the interview at their homes or at the community center next door. I conducted two interviews in a conference room at the Diabetes Wellness Center in Talihina. Many women preferred to participate in the interview on the day I recruited them, as they had already made the trip to pick up their commodities and driving back and forth could take hours. Picking up commodities is often considered an "all day" activity, so women often had only that engagement scheduled for the day and no other obligations until the evening. However, other women chose to make appointments with me on the following day, week, or next time I was in the area, which was sometimes the following month. Additionally, women often recommended names of friends or other community members they thought would be helpful for my research.[22] In all, I interviewed forty-nine women for this project, ranging from eighteen to seventy years of age, with the mean age being fifty-one years; the majority identified as "Choctaw only" (n = 42, 86 percent).[23] As the table shows, the women who shared their stories with me could be summarized as struggling with poverty, dependent on food assistance, living with compromised health, and considered to be "assimilated." At first glance, the women's narratives offer examples of lived experiences of the goal of settler colonialism, with poor health, poverty, and assimilation as means of elimination. However, this book will demonstrate that it is *within* this ongoing structure of settler colonialism where poor health, poverty, and assimilation have taken on new meanings and come to symbolize specific experiences of what it means to be Indigenous—experiences that have resulted in a collective solidarity and a point of departure for health initiatives.

The next chapter provides an intimate look at two women's food-centered life history narratives and situates actual stories within this context. I use their narratives as a stepping-off point for discussion throughout the book, as these stories (and one other presented later) were the most detailed narratives presented. By sharing these stories and using narrative data in multiple ways, I aim to demonstrate how the critical intersections between the experiences described in women's stories, the ways they make sense of them, obesity, and identity are fundamental to an embodied heritage framework of Indigenous health.

CHAPTER 2

Food and Fellowship

Intersections of Health, Violence, Trauma, and Indianness in Food-Centered Life Narratives

Food is a powerful voice, especially for those who are often heavily involved with its acquisition, preparation, provisioning, and cleanup (Hauck-Lawson 1998). Through close examinations of food narratives, researchers have found unique opportunities for understanding how people conceptualize and experience important historical, social, political and environmental factors affecting foods and foodways (Beauman et al. 2005; Bisogni et al. 2002; Counihan 1999; Sobal et al. 2006; Wansink 2004). These factors are best examined by exploring individuals' perceptions and meaning-making of food experiences in their everyday lives. I used food-centered life history narratives (Counihan 2002) to inquire into behaviors, experiences, beliefs, and memories centered on food production, preservation, preparation, consumption, distribution, and exchange. This method builds on the concept of *testimonios* (Bernal et al. 2012) as a way to bear witness and inscribe into history the lived realities of those most often silenced, erased, or voiceless.

As women spoke about food throughout this project, they revealed rich dimensions of their lives amid the rapidly changing social, cultural, and economic rural landscapes in which they live. Their stories, although anchored around food and foodways, speak to issues of poverty, trauma, violence, and simple survival, revealing individual subjectivity while calling attention to broad historical, political, and economic forces. The human relationship to food is complex and multidimensional: It biologically nourishes the body, culturally symbolizes belonging and love, and links individuals to the collective through psychological and social functions. The findings from these interviews with women reveal that food is indeed complex and multidimensional, as well as a medium to "getting at" larger social factors, so much so that it often felt that the more we talked about food, the less the conversation was about food. In other words, talking about food and foodways led to rich discussions about trauma, violence, relationality, and heritage.

This chapter uses women's food-centered life narratives to explore how historical trauma, contemporary violence, and identity intersect in ways that shape embodiment and heritage. These narratives illuminate the connections between obesity (and related conditions) and heritage, demonstrating how food stories can serve as powerful tools for articulating an embodied heritage framework. First comes Linda, a diabetic with severely compromised health who has endured a great deal of personal and social suffering, including poverty, racism, alcoholism, abandonment. Although in poor health herself, she became the primary caretaker of her grandson during her daughter's incarceration for drug-related crimes. Linda is known throughout the community and, even though she does not drive, is a constant presence at the local community center. Second is Sherry, an active woman who cares full-time for her dialysis-dependent sister, who recently suffered a stroke. At the age of eighteen, Sherry left her small rural hometown, moved to the city, studied data processing, and worked in various jobs until she retired. She is very active in her church and the surrounding community and is friendly and easy to talk to, but Sherry is haunted by trauma and shame. She is well-known for sewing traditional Choctaw dresses and is often hired by the Nation and cultural groups to make the dresses; this work gives her special insight into the changing sizes of Choctaw bodies. Both women have relied on government-issued commodity foods for as long as they can remember. Their food-centered life narratives illustrate key dimensions of historical trauma, violence, and the shaping of heritage and identity within an embodied heritage framework. Through their stories, this chapter reveals how multiple intersecting social forces underpin the lived experience of embodied heritage.

Linda's Story

Linda is a fifty-three-year-old Choctaw woman, born and raised in a one-room house on allotted land in "the country," the outskirts of a small, rural town at the foothills of the Kiamichi Mountains.[1] Her mother died young, leaving behind six children and a husband. Although not the oldest child, Linda became responsible for cooking, cleaning, and taking care of her siblings. At the age of sixteen, she moved away from home to live with two of her sisters in the nearest town, dropped out of high school, and got a job at a local chicken plant, where she worked for eighteen years. She is divorced, has three adult children, and is currently unemployed due to health reasons but remains the primary caregiver to her seven-year-old grandson.

We meet in a large, private room next to the cafeteria at the local community center and sit at tables where *Chahta anumpa* classes are taught. *Chahta* phrases and their English translations cover the whiteboard in front of us, and the fluorescent lights quietly hum above us. Linda, wearing a neon green t-shirt with pink daisies and the phrase "Oklahoma Girls Do It Right!" sits down across the table from me, looks me over and asks, "You Choctaw?" After situating me via my family name, she relaxes somewhat. We begin with the informed consent paperwork and then move on to the interview. Still not at ease, Linda sits stiffly with her purse strap taut around her shoulder.

"Yesterday morning, I ate an egg sandwich, and then I didn't eat nothing the rest of the day until supper. I ate nachos from the Mexican place . . ." Linda begins as she shifts her weight in the chair, softening a bit and letting the frayed purse strap fall off her shoulder. She continues, "I just scrambled [the egg] up and slapped it on the bread, put some ketchup on it, went and sat down, and ate it. That was it [chuckles]." At this point, she begins to relax, unwrapping the purse from her arm and setting it down on the table. She moves her hands up to the table, picks up a pen, and toys with it as she describes what a typical morning looks like in her home. Her grandson currently lives with her because his mom, Molly (who is Linda's oldest daughter), commutes to work in Arkansas at a chicken plant. "She comes and goes, but it's mainly me and him." Molly, who was recently released from prison, has been sober for two years. Her comings and goings are inconsistent and unpredictable, so Linda has been granted temporary guardianship of Molly's son.

Linda and I ease into the interview, talking about food and cooking, and she tells me that she likes to watch the Food Network on TV. Her favorite show is *Chopped*, and she explains, ". . . it's just how they can whip something up so fast with just a few ingredients. . . . I like to cook, but I don't cook nothing like that. I couldn't cook nothing they eat. Half the time, I can't pronounce what they saying, you know [chuckles]. I want to know what I'm eating, and I don't know what're the different ingredients in there.[2] I know it's hard to tell," Linda pauses and nods down toward her body,[3] ". . . but I'm a very picky person when it comes to food." Linda goes on to describe what she means by "picky": "I don't eat eggs cooked nowhere else, unless I cook it. I don't even eat it when my daughters cook it." She also uses "picky" to describe her experiences eating out. For example, she will not order or eat French fries from McDonald's, Arby's, or Sonic. Linda tells me that those fries, and food in general, just don't "taste right" anymore, and she attributes this to the multiple medications that she is taking for diabetes, high blood pressure and cholesterol, arthritis, and thyroid issues. When she first starts talking about her medications and what they're for, she rattles off, "Well, I have, of course, diabetes, high blood pressure, I guess you can say I'm a—they call me a heart patient. I have artificial valves, and so I take heart medicine, and then the thyroids. I take a thyroid therapy pill every day. Hopefully that was it [chuckles]. Just the regular stuff."

I am immediately aware of how Linda says, "I have, *of course,* diabetes . . ." (my emphasis), as well how she categorizes her health issues as "just the regular stuff," and ask her to elaborate on this. Like most of the women I interviewed, Linda links diabetes with being Native, describing it as an inevitable illness. "Because they said diabetes runs really bad in Native Americans, and that's just statistics." She continues, listing off family member after family member who has been diagnosed with diabetes: aunts and uncles; brothers and sisters; nieces and nephews; cousins, including a three-year-old cousin; even her own children.[4] When talking about her seventeen-year-old niece, she describes how she tries to warn youth about the dangers of diabetes.

> She's got type 2 diabetes real bad, real, really bad. And I try to talk to her. Because I know at that age, she's a teenager and she's not wanting to do

what she's supposed to do to take care of herself. And like I said, it's bad in the younger generation. . . . And diabetes, like I tell them [the younger generation] all the time, that's something you don't mess with. Diabetes is serious. I've had—I know a lot of people that lost a leg, or [went] blind, or kidneys, or something. I think diabetes is—they say it's really bad in the Native Americans, and I really believe it because I've seen it. I've lost a cousin years ago, and she was only like seventeen, eighteen, because of the kidney complication due to diabetes. I really do think that diabetes is something that's serious, and with Native Americans, because like I said, in my family, just in my family alone, I have seen it. I seriously think that's true. Diabetes is hereditary. That's one of the causes I know, because I've seen some that look like they're real healthy. They're not overweight or anything. I have a three-year-old cousin, he's a diabetic, because it ran in both sides. That's not even just how they eat and stuff. I know how you eat is one of the main issues . . . junk food, fried food.

Linda continues, telling me that she worries about her seven-year-old grandson, who weighs 110 pounds.

I think he was like three, four, and think he used food as comfort, and I let it happen because his mom was into drugs and got incarcerated for a whole bunch of stuff, and it was like, if he wanted something, it was easier to give [it] to him than deny him because of the situation he was going through, you know. Even if she wasn't in jail at that time, she was never home, never in his life. Just in and out, popping in and out. I think with him, I let him have that food[5] as comfort food if he was upset, and then he'd quit crying, and he'd want something. It was hard to deny him, because he was already hurt. I think that's why I worry about him and other kids.

Linda's concern for her grandson and other kids stems from her personal experiences and those she has witnessed among her friends and family members, many of whom are also grandmothers responsible full-time for their grandchildren. She worries first about her children's generation being "lost" to alcohol and drugs, poverty, lack of opportunities, and mistakes for which she holds her own generation responsible. Second, Linda worries about her grandchildren's generation, "lost" to obesity, diabetes, and addicted parents. Linda sighs deeply and returns to something she feels she *should* have more control over—junk foods and fried foods—

and comments, "Food that we like to eat, that we normally shouldn't. . . . It's hard to do when you're used to that life." As will become clearer, Linda's last sentence encompasses much more than just avoiding junk foods and fried foods. "It's hard to do when you're used to that life" references the constraints surrounding her individual agency, which is shaped by poverty, historical trauma, structural violence, and heritage.

Linda's CDIB card designates her as one-half Choctaw, but she tells me she is "full blood."[6] Under the fluorescent lights, her skin appears dark brown, especially noticeable in contrast to the neon green of her t-shirt. Her black hair, peppered with strands of white, sits at her shoulders, thick and unruly. She takes a drink of the water I had put out earlier and begins to tell me her story.

> My dad, he didn't have a roll number, that's why we're only considered half. I don't know if he came from Mississippi or if he was one of them Louisiana, Jena tribe, or the Coushatta, or something. I don't know what it was. He coulda been white, Black and whatever. I don't know. We didn't have no proof of what he was, but evidently, he was Choctaw because he spoke Choctaw. . . . My mom had a roll number, and that's where we got everything from. And my dad had land, and when they first started building the Indian homes, he told her she could get one, but she wouldn't get one.[7] I don't know what was wrong with my mom either, I always say she was crazy. Now that I'm older, I guess I can see—to us, it was actually, in today's age it would have been abuse, because of the way, you know, I was slapped, I had my hair pulled, and hit with her cane, and everything else. But now I try to look at it as, when I'm older now, that she couldn't do the things—that maybe she felt like she's not doing the things she's supposed to be doing for us. Instead, we was doing for her. And we was bathing her and everything. At only eight, nine, ten years old. That wasn't our place to do it.[8]

Linda was only twelve when her mother, cripped and bedridden from severe rheumatoid arthritis, died at the age of forty. For the last three years of her mother's life, Linda acted as her primary caregiver. She continues:

> She needed to be either in a home or have a nurse come and check on her or something. But we had to take up that slack. I remember a time when

I stood over the kitchen stove. I probably was about nine years old. I was tryin' to cook eggs—*I guess I'm like her*—tryin' to cook eggs to her liking, and each time I took it to her, it wasn't right, and I got hit. And I don't even know what happened [after that]. I never knew what happened. Did she ever eat? How did I quit cooking the eggs? Did she knock me out? Now that I look back I can—and then I have images, like sometimes my sisters and I will sit around and talk, "I kind of remember that," you know. Just a flashback but it wasn't a—you know, I hear a lot of people talk about their mothers, how they used to do this. My sister-in-law lost her mother two years ago. She talks about "Mom this," "Mom that." And we was talking one day, and I said, "Yeah, I don't have no memories, not no good memories of my mother," and that's sad. And I don't want my kids to be like that. [emphasis added][9]

Linda's mother was forced to attend a boarding school as a child, but Linda does not know any of the details. Her mother never spoke about it, and Linda is not even sure which of the schools she attended. All she knows is that she did go to a boarding school, and they never discussed it.

That's why I say, I don't know nothing about [my parents]. My dad, he was the only child and his parents, I barely remember them. They passed on, like I said. I was young. I barely remember them, and dad didn't have no siblings so his family just, like, died out. I don't know nothing about them. And my mom . . . yeah.[10]

Linda shrugs her shoulders, sighs deeply, and looks down. Like many of the women I have spoken with, she carries an emptiness. It is a palpable emptiness that comes from not knowing family histories; knowing only key notes, but no details; not knowing what to tell her own children about where they come from, who they are, how to speak their language; and an emptiness from not trusting what they *do* know (or what they think they know, or how they know what they know).

Linda's father died from a massive heart attack at the age of seventy-two, alone in the one-room house on their allotted land. Linda was well into adulthood at the time of his death, but she still reports not knowing much about him, not ever getting to really know him. Our conversation moves fluidly back and forth through time, as Linda describes her childhood.

> I grew up in a rough life. Really rough. Compared to others, my kinfolks my age, I seen them, I mean, they all pretty much grew up in more modern times than us. . . . We grew up poor. I guess you would say we was dirt poor. I was still in high school, and we didn't even have electricity. We didn't have running water. Everybody else did. We didn't. There was all eight of us in a little one-room house. One big room. We had a bed in one corner, and that's how we slept. Growing up, it wasn't as—it didn't bother us, I guess. Some of my sisters said they had kids make fun of them because maybe our clothes smelled dirty . . . and as I got older, I remember telling a lot of little white lies just to—you know, kids be talking about what they watched on TV, and they'd say, "Did you watch it?" I was like, "No, I went to my grandpa's house." It was, like, embarrassing as I got older. At the younger age I guess it didn't bother me. I remember being picked on at school a few times. It was like some of them didn't want to be my friend, maybe because of the way I looked, the way I dressed. I don't know. I wouldn't wish that on anybody else. . . .
>
> Every day, we ate beans and rice, fried potatoes, and biscuits. That was our meal every day, every week, day-in, day-out. I don't know if that's all my dad could afford or that was just what we ate. And, of course, my dad—we had chickens, well, he'd go out there and wring a neck or two, and that's all we ate. . . . On Fridays, I think, when my dad got paid, he might've brought us some Kool-Aid or something, but we didn't really have a lot of sweets or nothing. I guess it was all that rice [that caused the diabetes]. We lived on rice. I mean, we ate rice. To this day, that's all my family knows is rice. Just white rice. Just boiled, white rice. Then I come to find out that's one of the worst things for a diabetic. But like I tell my dietician, I thought I was doing good because rice, I boil it in water. No salt, no grease, nothing.[11]

When I first meet Linda, she is visibly suffering from health issues. Her skin is dull and lusterless; her eyes, tight with pain and glazed; and her chest heaves up and down, seemingly fighting for constricted breaths. She moves slowly, but not necessarily deliberately. Illness is a large part of Linda's life now. Her general health is very poor—as she describes in our interview but also as calculated from one of the surveys she completes about daily life and activities—matching her narrative and appearance. She reports severe limitations in physical functioning, energy, and physical pain. Continuing to combine an explanatory model of diet and exercise with a fatalistic viewpoint regarding diabetes, Linda explains to me:

> I guess, since they say Native Americans get diabetes faster, I guess we eat more than what we should, or at least that's what it would be, but I don't really see no difference in the food. It's just how a person eats it. And your body, I guess. But then, like I said, if it's hereditary, and I know diabetes is, but I guess it would just depend on how you eat, or whether you eat. You're going to be healthy or not, and that's the good Lord's will. . . .[12] I was never this big. Before I had my surgery, I probably weighed 110, 120 [pounds]. But I know a lot of mine now is not exercising, and with the thyroid problem, that's a lot of mine, and since I'm not working, there's days I don't do nothing. There's days I don't have no energy. I can sleep all day. But then at night, I'm restless, and a lot of mine is anxiety.

Here, Linda pauses, squints her eyes, and says quietly (which initially seems disconnected to me):

> Or like they say, "You can tell they're Choctaws, they're drunk," or "Must have been a Choctaw," if something's happening and you read in the papers, something to do with alcoholism, "I bet that was a Choctaw," you know. Why? Other people drinks too. But most of the time, it's Native Americans [chuckles]. Just here a while back, one of the stores got broken into. They stole some beer. They was trying to identify the person, and they said, "I bet it was a Choctaw. You know them." The only thing they stole is beer. They didn't get nothing else, just beer. I thought, you know, why you think it's got to be a Choctaw? Then they say, "Choctaws get drunk all the time." Alcohol, right there. It ties with the Native Americans, and diabetes ties with the Native Americans. That shouldn't be no big issue over that, because alcoholism is in everybody, not just Native Americans. Diabetes, too. I guess it happens with Native Americans more, maybe that's why.[13]

Linda weaves her personal experiences of anxiety, diabetes, and alcoholism throughout our conversation. She tells me that she struggled with alcoholism, but it is clearly a painful subject for her, difficult to talk about. She hangs her head shamefully, and her brow furrows as she tells me first about her daughter, Molly.

> She and I has been through a lot, but she has straightened up. I think she's been sober for two years now. She was into drugs, bad. She was shooting up and stealing and all, I guess to support her habit. And she went to jail for that. She had drugs on her, pills on her, all the whatever, she—they found needles and everything. She wasn't at home then. She was staying with a friend, and I had [Molly's son]. And then she went to jail, served her time, I think she stayed in there like six months, got out on probation, still wouldn't listen, still didn't straighten up, went back to jail, got out, went back to jail, got out, and at that point, one of my other daughters had temporary guardianship over [Molly's son], because I didn't—they told me I couldn't try for guardianship with my health issue and stuff.

She pauses here, shrugs and looks forlornly at the table before continuing to tell me that Molly began using drugs while still in high school; she then stopped going to high school, and Linda really struggled to help Molly get sober, to no avail. Finally, she kicked Molly out of the house, and shortly thereafter, Molly found out she was pregnant.

> Then when she got pregnant, of course she came home, and I let her come home. And I had told her she can come back home. I had told her, "After you have the baby," I said, "I'm going to quit working and stay home and take care of the baby, you go to work and take care of me. I've been working years to take care of y'all." Well, it didn't work out that way. What worked out was, that's when I got sick and ended up having open-heart surgery. At the same time, she had [the baby], I was in the hospital, and I had just come home on Monday, and that following Monday she had him. And then he got airlifted out to Little Rock . . . and he didn't come home for three months.

Linda doesn't elaborate on her grandson's health, why he had to be airlifted out of state, or why he didn't come home for three months, but she continues to tell me about Molly.

I guess, I don't know, I think she had, uh, how would you say it? When she was born, she had a cleft lip, bi-lateral, and I don't think she was, like, real, um, feels secure about her looks, or, I don't know. I think sometimes she had that issue, and because she blamed me for a lot of things, which is, I know, typical for teenagers, you know. "You done it." I say, "Yes, I know I done that." Because I used to drink a lot. I did when they were younger. By the time their dad and I split up, of course, I started drinking. And that alcoholism, like I said, that's another major issue for Native Americans. It's sad, but I've seen it in my family. I done it, and well, that was the reason why—that was the reason for our divorce. But after our divorce, I done the same thing. Yeah, and I done it for years. My girls, they were little, but for some reason she never blamed her dad for nothing. I guess it's because they stayed with me. It was easier to blame me, and she just got worse and worse and got into—the kids she hung around with, I know it wasn't their fault, but her friends, they all done the same thing. She just went from drinking to smoking marijuana and then into the—because at that time I didn't know she was shooting up or anything. . . . But I think that's—she just went through a lot. And she still does. We still fight like cats and dogs whenever she's around. I think that's what it is; diabetes and alcoholism is really bad in Native Americans. And it's sad to say, but I just seen it happen in my family over and over. And not only family but with friends, too.

Linda lists all the family members and friends she has lost from alcoholism: aunts and uncles, brothers and sisters, cousins, her children, and so on. Her ticking off family members who suffer from alcoholism is eerily similar to the list of family members with diabetes she shared earlier.

I've seen them go through the same thing, you know, to where—and any of us, we don't drink no more. None of my brothers or sisters drink anymore, but you know we've all done it. And I've seen all my cousins because we all done it together so it's like—it's just there, just like diabetes. It's just there. Hereditary, I guess. I don't know if alcohol is or not, but it seemed like it would be. Because I've seen it, with the diabetes and then, when I look back, I could see the alcohol there, too, right along with that diabetes. You know?

I ask Linda why she thinks diabetes and alcohol are hereditary in Native Americans, and interestingly, she begins to talk about "being Indian." At first, I think maybe she didn't understand my question, but it quickly becomes clear to me that she is weaving the lack of a clear, congruent Choctaw identity and cultural dispossession into her explanatory model of diabetes and alcohol among Natives.

> We grew up, we wouldn't, it wasn't like we knew. We just—I don't know, growing up, I don't know if I ever looked at myself as Indian, or what. I's just, me. My dad and mom, they spoke Choctaw. But I don't know it. I mean I understand it. I might put few words together, but just to sit here and speak it? No. But I understand it. I don't know if *that* [loss of language] had anything to do with *that* [high rates of diabetes and alcoholism].[14] Like I said, they spoke it, but they didn't make us speak it. Dad never took us to any cultural things. I didn't know anything about that until of course I was in high school and then started going to powwows then. But I'm not into that stuff. I don't care for powwows. I just don't. I go to church. I like to go to church singings. That I'll go, but anything else. . . .

Linda trails off at this point, saying she doesn't like to attend most of the "cultural stuff" because of her health issues, but more importantly, because it is unfamiliar. To Linda, as well as most of the older women I spoke to, the cultural events available to the youth today are unrecognizable. They express not being sure whether these cultural events or gatherings just were not "out there" when they were young, or if there had been such events but they just didn't attend; at any rate, today's powwows, dances, storytelling, stickball, and other events seem "new" to them. Even *Chahta anumpa* as taught by the Choctaw Nation is unfamiliar to some of these women. Although Linda says she doesn't speak *Chahta*, when I first met her, she was speaking in *Chahta* to an older woman at the community center. At one time during the interview, she also nodded to the whiteboard in the room and read aloud the *Chahta* sentences, remarking, "I wish my kids had learned to speak Choctaw because now all that language stuff is going away. Well, they're teaching it now, so they're trying to bring it back, but it's different from how we grew up, from what we heard; it's worded different."[15]

Like Linda, several other women who participated in this project told me that the *Chahta anumpa* the Nation is teaching to the wider community is much different than what they grew up hearing and speaking. Many of them pointed out differences in both vocabulary and structure, which led a couple of them to hypothesize that the language curriculum developers at the Choctaw Nation were maybe teaching Mississippi *Chahta anumpa* (rather than Oklahoma *Chahta*). But the majority of the women I spoke with internalized these noted differences as their own lack of knowledge, ability, or improper language usage, not trusting what they know; thus, many of them claimed to not "know" *Chahta* (regardless of the fact that many of them speak it daily with each other).

Linda tells me that she is trying to teach her grandson *Chahta*—just a few simple words—but she laments:

> I don't know . . . he use words, and he don't know if he's saying it in Choctaw, Spanish, or what because his grandpa—my ex-husband—is Mexican. And he don't know. He [my grandson] don't know if he's Indian. He don't know if he's Mexican . . . and that's just words we grew up saying. He's the same way, he don't know if it, "Is that Mexican like my papa says or is it Choctaw like us?" And he don't know, he'll say, "Am I Choctaw or am I Mexican?" But I don't know. I don't know.

My conversation with Linda ends shortly after this, with the unknowingness of how her grandson will grow to identify himself. This question of "who are we" is an important one for Choctaws, raised in interview after interview and throughout the ethnography of this research. Heritage is an essential component of an embodied heritage framework that will be explored in depth in later chapters, but the important point here is that Linda has identified a double bind of Choctaw identity in these moments: A distinct cultural identity is needed upon which Choctaws can claim rights and recognition, yet it is an identity that is currently being co-created alongside the demand for distinction. Thus, expressions of that identity (e.g., *Chahta anumpa* classes, cultural events) seem unfamiliar, can feel inauthentic, and at the very least make these women question what they know about *being* Choctaw.

Like the other women I interviewed, Linda's story focused mostly on diabetes, rather than obesity. This is perhaps because they were able to talk more explicitly about diabetes. Diabetes is widely and consistently recognized as a disease. The Nation has focused extensively on diabetes, making available diabetes-related devices (e.g., shoes, walking devices, care plans, nutritionists, specific classes, etc.) and diabetes clinics. It also widely advertises diabetes-related events, issues, topics, etc. Obesity, while also recognized as a disease in medicine and public health, is largely internalized among these women (and also promoted by the Nation) as an individual behavior or lifestyle choice, even though many of them recognize its historical origins and link it with limited access to healthy foods. Furthermore, obesity is widespread and not visibly/directly related to outcomes like amputation, blindness, or dialysis (even though most recognize the linkage of obesity with diabetes), and finally, being "chubby" is seen as healthy and generally harmless.

Linda's story mirrored others' stories in this research, where there were fluid interactions between health status, obesity, historical trauma, poverty, structural violence, and cultural identity. What stands out to me from Linda's story (and so many others') is the normalization of suffering and disease, what Nancy Scheper-Hughes (1993) calls *everyday violence.* Linda normalized her compromised health as "just the regular stuff." As I listened to Linda's words and later reviewed the transcript, this statement stuck with me and made me think about the very ordinary linkage of contemporary violence and disease. That is, how Linda (and many of the other women in this project) biologizes and racializes diabetes (and alcoholism) and how the alarming number of people she knows who are suffering with these two conditions is not to be seen as alarming at all, but rather as normal among Choctaws and "to be expected."

Although subtly, Linda situates her diabetes within a wider range of variables, including material and cultural dispossession, trauma, inequality, and emotional suffering. In the book *Hard Earned Lives: Accounts of Health and Illness from East London,* Jocelyn Cornwell (1984:15−6) identifies a dichotomy between "public accounts" as "sets of meanings in common social currency that reproduce and legitimate the larger assumptions people hold about the nature of social reality" and "private accounts" which "spring directly from personal experience and from the thoughts and feelings accompanying it." Linda's account illustrates Cornwell's observation that answers to specific prompts tend to invite a "public account," and she often referred to a larger collective of "Native Americans" (note her usage of "*the* Native American"), drawing on themes of historical change and disenfranchisement. By contrast, Linda's own storytelling results in a more "private account," where she discloses specific details and circumstances that reveal her personal linkages of alcoholism and diabetes with anxiety and trauma.

Sherry's Story

Sherry is a sixty-nine-year-old Choctaw woman, proud that she never married or had children of her own and invested much of her life in working and participating in Indian church. She lives alone in the second largest city on the reservation but grew up on allotted land in the mountains, right in the heart of Choctaw country and not too far from where she lives now. Her family's land was a large farm located in the valley, a sandy loam surrounded by native pine and home to whitetail deer, turkeys, wild hogs, dove, and quail. At eighteen, Sherry graduated high school and left to work at a sewing factory in the city. She relocated multiple times thereafter, searching for better work opportunities, and ended up in Oklahoma City, where she spent most of her years working at various locations and in multiple roles: a sewing factory, a data processing center, the state health department, a police department, a power company, and finally a chemical company, post-retirement. Sherry is more economically secure than the majority of the women interviewed for this project. She has worked all her life and has a sufficient retirement fund. Her sister has recently had a stroke, so Sherry has returned to care for her.

In at least three interviews with other women, Sherry's name has come up as a key person to include in this research. She is a constant figure at her local church, the community center, and the weekly senior lunches, and she is a very talented dressmaker, well known across the Nation, her dresses worn by Choctaw singers, royalty, and other cultural groups, as well as by everyday women. She is very active, keeps herself busy, and is highly regarded within the community. We meet in the early afternoon on a weekday at the community center, and Sherry has just come from church, where she and four other women have voluntarily mowed the lawn. Each week in the warm months, she meets her friends there to cut the grass while another woman cooks them a breakfast of bacon, eggs, and biscuits and gravy in the church's kitchen. At 5'2" and 189 pounds, Sherry is a solid, strong woman with white curly hair that frames her round face, darkened from her time spent outdoors. She is jovial, smiling, and jokes with me immediately. She asks if I am Native, and nods with a smile when I tell her my father is Choctaw and my mother is *nahullo* (white).[16]

Sherry, like most of the women in this research who relocated to cities for jobs or other opportunities, has returned home to care for family members. Her entire family is diabetic, and her sister and nephew are on dialysis. Sherry, who is not diabetic, only began to consider her own health once she moved back: "After I moved down here—like I say, my whole family has diabetes, so I do take the test regular to make sure." Other than being categorized as clinically obese on the Body Mass Index (BMI), Sherry has no other health issues and reports her health as "good."[17] We jump right into talking about food, diabetes, and health.

> I think the biggest change is in processed food. . . . It's just because, we grew up where we raised everything. I just didn't see as much sickness when I was growing up as I see now. Young people are sick or diabetic. I think it's the foods. . . . Everybody is saying they're diabetic and if they get hurt, like a wound, it won't heal. I don't know. It's just really rampant among our Indian people.

Sherry takes a deep breath here, steadying herself, and begins to describe what it was like when her sister was diagnosed with diabetes.

> To me it was bad, but to her, like most Indian people, it doesn't really faze them when they say, "You've got diabetes." It's just, they expect it. "Well, I've got diabetes," and that's it. It does not make them want to do better, change your ways or anything. I think that they consider that diabetes is an Indian disease. They think, "Well, if I'm Indian I'm going to get it. It's just a matter of when," because probably everybody you know, almost, has it . . . same with obesity. I think Indian people, they're just not really, they're really not that much concerned about their health. If it happens, it happens; and if it don't, it don't.

Sherry recognizes this fatalistic perspective of diabetes and obesity as common among Indian people that Linda (and so many other women

I spoke with) expressed: Indians are going to get diabetes because they are Indian, so why bother? Sherry notes, "I have non-Native friends that when they're told they have diabetes, they go on a diet. They lose the weight, they eat right. I don't see the Indians doing that. I guess *it is* like an Indian disease [chuckles]."[18]

I understand Sherry's last sentence, "I guess *it is* like an Indian disease," to mean, rather than that diabetes is an "Indian disease," that it is, instead, the indifferent, fatalistic perspective of diabetes among Indians that is actually the "Indian disease." This is an important distinction, and Sherry elaborates further.

> Watching my sister, of course—she's—like I said, she doesn't seem to take it seriously. She still goes ahead and does things the doctors tell her not to. It causes blindness, and she's eventually—over time, she's lost her eyesight. She barely sees now. It's like, "Well, so what?" She is on dialysis. . . . I try to get her to walk. I say, "If you just walk around in the yard, just around the house." And she's, "But I don't want to." They just want to sit, and her son is the same way. They just want to sit and watch TV or sleep. They won't try to get up and walk around or anything. . . . I don't know if it's self-respect, maybe low self-esteem, that it's like they expect these things to happen in that order. "It's going to happen, so I'm not going to do anything about it."

The issues of self-respect, low self-esteem, and shame are important to Sherry. The rest of our conversation centers around these feelings, which are central tenets of Sherry's explanatory model of why obesity and diabetes are rampant among Natives.

> I think it dates way back. [Indians] feel like they are not as good as the next person. Of course, there's a lot of people that make them feel that way. "Well, I'm Indian, I'll never make anything. I'll never be anything." They don't even try. They kind of just say, "Well, you know, it happens." I was not sent to a boarding school, but I have friends that were. They say they were not allowed to speak the language. They were not allowed to be Indian. I don't think it is just there [at the boarding schools], and it's still . . .[19]

Sherry pauses here, her voice trembles, and she describes a painful experience at the First Baptist Church in Oklahoma City, illustrating the ways in which people are *still* not allowed to be Indian. In her telling, white church members said to her, "There's a church on the hill for your type of people." She tells me in detail:

> They don't want [Indians] coming to their churches. They'll direct you to the Indian church. . . . They say everybody's equal, but this is not true. I go to a country church, that's where I grew up, but we have white people that come. Their main thing is they want to change the Indian to their [white] way. They think we're so far back that we need them to come and show us how to worship. . . . I think that's why the Indian has low self-esteem, because they're always put down. It's sad when it's our churches that's put them down.[20]

At this point, Sherry begins sobbing, tears stream down her face, and she hunches over in pain. I don't have any tissues in this borrowed office, so I run to the restroom and unroll streams of toilet paper. I bring it back to her to wipe her tears, apologizing for bringing her toilet paper, and we begin to laugh at the strangely intimate moment that passes between us. Sherry and I look at each other, both of us teary and laughing at the bunched-up toilet paper. She apologizes for crying and continues, now telling me about her brother.

> It's just that my own brother is married to a white, and she tries to change him. She *has* changed him. He does not claim to be Indian unless there's a benefit for him.[21] It hits home when we see all that. They're always saying that the Indian does not know what they're doing. I guess it hurts more when it's the churches that are doing this. They're always trying to bring their ways into church. Basically, I think that the Indian is more spiritual than the other non-Indians because, to [Indians], everything is sacred. [Indians] don't go out and kill wild animals other than for food. [Indians] don't cut down trees for lumber unless they need it. These are the things that I see, even in our little country church down there, they think that, and they come in and tell us, "You need to do this, you need to do that." We've been here a lot longer than they have.[22]

She chuckles at her own comment, and after a long pause, and without further explanation, Sherry states directly, "I don't like to read history of the Indian, like the Trail of Tears. I don't like hearing a thing about that because I really get sick. If it was just left alone—I realize it's in the past, and our people came through it, but they don't leave it alone. It comes up all the time."

Sherry's insight into the way that history constantly resurfaces is accurate. Across towns on the reservation, tropes of "cowboys and Indians" and the Trail of Tears canvas buildings, murals, signs, and events. Much of the recalling is done as a remembrance or in commemoration, like the Nation's annual Trail of Tears Walk, but sometimes the past is called upon in incredibly painful ways.[23] I understand Sherry's comment, however, to mean that the past is not that far away. That is, the pain is still present, it is still present in our bodies, and our struggles and experiences are still connected with it. The past—especially the trauma and violence associated with it—is not far enough removed yet to commemorate it without feeling it. This is particularly interesting, because Sherry does not sit in a place of victimhood; she does not consider herself or other Choctaws as victims. Rather, she still feels the pain of past traumatic events in the present, and for her, this is what is making people sick. Further, she worries about the younger generation because she sees this repeated as everyday violence.

> I don't know that it's getting worse. I think they have different angles that they come at the young people with. I hear parents tell their kids or grandkids, "Don't hang around with that person. I don't want you to hang around with those Indians," or, "You're acting like an Indian, like a wild Indian" when they get rowdy, or stuff like that that you hear. I think it sticks with our young people. They just use languages that maybe they're don't thinking anything about it. Maybe they do, I don't know. These young people, they have a hard time in school. Anything that they say against the Indian is going to stick with them.

Sherry is choked up again, visibly distraught, and we pause for a moment. I ask her if she'd like to keep going, and she nods yes, drinks some water, and steers the conversation toward obesity-related issues. "I've heard young people say that 'I probably didn't get the job because I'm too fat.' They're looking at their self-image, and because that person was tall, skinny, blond, they were the ones that got the job."

Sherry is describing the employment landscape of the Choctaw Nation, the largest employer in the region. During my participant observation, I also noted how many of the employees in various roles were non-Native, and in conversations with Choctaws, several described difficulty in getting a job with the Nation. For example, most of the jobs available at the time were night shifts at the casinos or travel plazas, and those with children and families to care for could not work overnight hours. Others described not being able to secure reliable transportation to get to places of employment. On the other hand, Sherry associates obesity with this disparity. "In a job, most people want people who can get around faster. Overweight people can't. It's a drawback, but what do we do about it? We're overweight. Until we get to the point that we want to better ourselves and lose weight and be more healthy, we're not going to be there."

Sherry goes on to say that "laziness" is what is preventing people from losing weight and being healthier and, showcasing herself as example, contradicts herself, illustrating the powerful internalization of obesity as a simple lifestyle or behavioral problem.

> Every day I say I'm going to start losing weight and haven't done it yet. It's hard to lose weight. I think, of course, the older you get the less exercise you do, so you're not going to lose weight. . . . I don't sit around and do nothing. Like I said, mowing this morning, and I mow my yard, and my sister's yard, and just do all that. I don't lay around, I don't watch TV, but I can't lose weight.

Among the women who participated in this research, Sherry is by far the most active, physically and socially. Although she is heavy and has a head full of white hair, her body is solid, strong, and she appears at least fifteen years younger than her almost seventy years. It is also interesting how Sherry shifts back and forth from blaming individuals (Choctaws) for being "fat and lazy" to critically identifying structural violence and historical trauma as key to current poor health among Choctaws. Further, she describes the cultural phenomenon between obesity and Natives as "Indians like to eat."

> I'm heavier right now than I've ever been. I don't know what to do other than quit eating and, of course, Indians like to eat. They like the fellowship,

and our churches, I was telling the pastor the other day, I said, "The only way I'm going to lose weight is to quit goin' to church" [laughter]. He said, "You can't do that," but every time you turn around, they're eating. And, well, you know, self-will, because only you can change that. . . . I think it's a tradition that Indian people, they like to share what they have, and they like to eat, and they want someone to eat with them. I think it brings them closer together. By sharing, by eating, by fellowshipping. They can't fellowship unless they're eating [laughter]. It does bring them close together.[24]

Sherry describes how, every Sunday, church members participate in a potluck, noting that "once it gets to the church on the table, it's not your food anymore. It's everybody's food." Important here are the acts of sharing food, eating together, and being together. I visited Sherry's church and potluck lunch; people brought all kinds of foods, in huge quantities: fried chicken, fried okra, macaroni salad, green beans, meatloaf, fried potatoes, hominy, and salt meat. Each person had a Styrofoam plate with dividers for three spaces to separate different foods. No one took only three foods, however; they filled the plates with each food item available, piling their plates up high. Food pushed over the edges of the raised plate dividers, the plates creasing, bending with each new food plopped atop the others; plates were pushed to their breaking point from the weight of the foods. The eating and fellowshipping lasted several hours, much longer than the actual church service did, and few leftovers remained. Churchgoers encouraged each other to "get full" and continuously asked, "Jeet yet?" ("Did you eat yet?") to gauge if someone was full. When newcomers entered, in addition to a greeting of "Hello, how are you?" they were asked, "Jeet yet? Grab a plate and get yourself something to eat!"

The weekly church potluck consists of mostly Southern foods. Sherry tells me that they used to have Choctaw foods at their potlucks, but that has been pushed to their annual "Indian day," the once a year Singing when they sing in *Chahta anumpa.*

[The service] used to be in Choctaw. It was. It was always an Indian church, but we threw off the "Indian" part because most of the people are non-Indian. We're losing our language. We're losing our culture. It's just a church now. It's still known as "the Indian Church," but we don't do the things that they used to do as Indian people. . . . Each generation gets away

from it. Right now, our Indian kids have married into whites, so we're losing the Indian. My sister and I are the only two Indians out there [in her
family] that you can say are Indian. The rest of them might have a little
drop of blood, but it's, it's . . . we've lost it.[25]

Our conversation moves back to obesity, and like many of the other
women, Sherry finds humor in her own big body. She jokes about eating too much, having a big appetite, and she enjoys teasing and being
teased by relatives and close friends—other Indians. Commenting on
one's weight and how much they eat is often done in an endearing way; it
is a dynamic and fun exchange of teasing among and within community.
Sherry explains:

> My nephew calls me "the short fat woman" [laughter]. The thing about it is,
> it does not bother me for an Indian to say it to me, but for someone else to
> say it to me, it irritates me. Because we're all in the same boat, basically . . .
> and we all like to kid each other. But don't let somebody else come in and
> try to kid you [laughter]. We understand what our joking is, but the outside
> does not understand. [A non-Indian] could say the same thing to me that
> some Indian said to me, and it would be all wrong because of who they
> were [laughter]. See? That's why I say Indians understand each other and
> they know when you mean it and when you don't. A non-Indian can say
> the very same thing, and I don't know if it's the tone of voice or what, but
> it gets to you.

Explaining obesity, Sherry tells me "There are medical things that
cause it," like, for example, thyroid problems, but her opinion is, "A lot
of it is not being able to afford the food that is healthy." She begins to
speak about the commodity foods program, noting the limits around
fresh foods but also tapping into something that is not fully discussed in
scholarly literature: taste preference for unhealthy foods among Indians.

> I think it's better now than it used to be, but I think there could be some
> improvement there. More fresh vegetables. On the other hand, a lot of
> Indians don't like fresh vegetables. I don't know. My sister doesn't like
> vegetables, period. She'll eat sweets, she'll eat chips, and stuff like that,
> but she doesn't want vegetables. . . . I think that's what she said, was that

"well I had to eat it when I was a kid because we didn't have anything else, you know." If you didn't eat what was on the table, then you didn't eat. And she said, "Well I had to eat it when I was a kid, so I don't have to eat it now because I am grown up." So, she eats what she wants. . . . We ate a lot of corn because we grew up in the country, on a farm. There was times we didn't have food other than corn that we raised. It was cooked every which way it could be cooked: ground for cornmeal, I mean cornbread, boiled, fried, or roasted, or whatever it is, it was corn [laughter], sometimes three times a day. That was pretty much it, other than Sundays. We always had neighbors over to eat with us, even though we didn't have a whole lot. That's when mom would kill a chicken and have fried chicken. What I remember most is that we had to wait 'til the last. The visitors ate first, so we usually got the wings.

Sherry's family also received government food assistance when she was a kid—it was not through the Choctaw Nation—and she recalls that it was often old and infested with bugs. (This was mentioned by several other women, and one told me the bug infestations in these foods were why her family fried foods all the time.)

I can remember Mom and them gettin' peanut butter, and that powdered milk, and cornmeal, and stuff like that, but it was all—a lot of it was buggy when they got it because it was old. . . . Yes, it was old stuff. . . . I mean, you would get cornmeal that had weevils in it and stuff. Canned goods were way outdated. . . . And that's why I say it's better now than it used to be, but I don't know. I think there's a lot of stuff to think and do differently.[26]

One of those things to do differently, according to Sherry, is to set a blood quantum cut-off limit for Choctaws. Specifically, because there seems to be too many people claiming to be Indian just so they can receive benefits, like commodity foods or healthcare. Sherry is deeply conflicted: She has an internalized shame of being Indian that is prevalent among her generation, but she also recognizes the beauty and tradition of her culture and identity. She also describes her family as being torn apart because her brother married a *nahullo* who, Sherry explained, prevents her brother from "acting Indian." This taps into the shame that Sherry carries.

A lot of people are not—they don't want to be Indian unless there's a benefit for them. And if you'll notice, since it started, Choctaw tags, everybody in [city] has a Choctaw tag.[27] And these are people who don't claim to be an Indian until there's something for them. . . . I think oh, well you say you don't want to be Indian, or you don't want to be around Indians, yet you know . . . so it kind of lowers your standard. Even though I don't say, "Well, you know you're doing this," but I just think that they shouldn't be cashing in on the benefits if they don't want to be Indian. . . . I think and I see this, like I said, my own brother is this way, but their spouse has a lot to do with it, because he doesn't say, "I'm not Indian." He just does not want to be around Indians—they have no Indian friends, and yet he's Indian. And if he want something, of course he goes to the clinic and all that, then he's Indian! And she [brother's wife] wants him to be Indian because he can go to the clinic and hospital and all that. But other than that, they don't hang around any Indian people. I think if they can't stand up and say, "I'm Choctaw," or "I'm Indian," then . . . that's in my own family so that's why I say it's—I see it![28]

Our conversations shifts back to obesity again, and Sherry, who has made Choctaw dresses for several years, has a unique vantage point on how Choctaw bodies have changed over time. She tells me about her experiences with dressmaking and the ways traditional dresses are changing.

I'm making more bigger dresses now than I used to. I used to make girl's [dresses], and they were slim, maybe a size twelve, fourteen or something like this, pretty much. There were some bigger sizes, but now I'm getting into the twenties and twenty-fours. . . . [I have to] get more material, and when [the girls are] slim, the dresses look better because they have more gathering in [them], because [the girls are] smaller. But then when you get a bigger person—like last night, I measured one lady, she was sixty-four inches around her waist. Well, that means that your material is forty-four inches wide, so she's not going to have much gathers in hers, so [laughs]. But I see that, and it seem like, that in this year, that the majority of my dresses have been [size] sixteen on up.

Sherry describes the structure of a Choctaw dress: It is designed to fit in the shoulders and then gather tightly at the waist, held together with a decorated waistband and apron. The smaller the person's waist is, the more gathering of cloth there will be at the waist. Thus, the bigger the person's waist is, the less gathering there will be. She tells me:

> In fact, some of them are going to be more like a muumuu rather than having a waist. Because [these girls] are heavy! And they got this [belly] roll like I got [laughter], so you don't even need a waist band! . . . See, I make these dresses, but I don't have one myself because I see how they look on heavier women. . . . I enjoy doing them for the little girls and the skinny women because you got a lot of gathers, and it looks good. But the heavier women, it just, and I just—sometimes I think, well I'm just going to start just making up to certain size, but then most of my clients, they're big women, so . . .

Our conversation winds down at this point, and I ask Sherry if there is anything else she would like to add. She again mentions how Choctaws are losing culture and traditions, specifically respect for elders.

> Young people have no respect for elders, they have no respect for any-thing. . . . I guess my biggest thing about Indian culture is respect for older people, because I see that the kids don't, and we try to teach our kids at church respect, "Respect those elder people." They're not taught at home. That is the one thing, because I've been to a lot of these—they call them senior gatherings, senior—whatever, but then there's a lot of kids there, and if there's food, they cut in line in front of the seniors. Well, if it's a senior program, the seniors need to be there. But a lot of these people bring their grandkids, and [the kids] don't show respect, and they'll push an old senior out the way and get up front. And I see that, and those are the things I think that if we could correct and train our young people, be a lot more respect.

I ask her what she thinks about how the Choctaw Nation is offering language classes and other things around culture. Sherry, like many of the other women in this project, tells me:

> The language classes? I've tried, and then I dropped out because I couldn't learn it. . . . My grandma spoke it all the time, and then when I went to

this language class the words were different. It's a modern thing, I guess. These people that are translating our study books, they're younger people, so they're using modern stuff. That was the other thing that, I couldn't just really get into it because I thought, this is not really Choctaw. I wanted to learn, and the teacher, she spoke the real Choctaw, but then she was having to go by the book. She would say a word, or someone would say a word in Choctaw. Well, I've heard my grandma talk enough of it that I knew it wasn't right. I mean it wasn't being pronounced right. It was difficult for me, so I just could not understand it.[29]

Embodied Heritage Framework

These two stories illuminate how historical trauma; structural, symbolic, and everyday violence; heritage and identity; and obesity and diabetes intersect. First, historical trauma is a constant presence in each woman's story through erased histories, boarding schools that practiced systematic cultural dispossession (i.e., loss of language and traditional cultural expressions), and shaken epistemologies that present as distrust in what one knows about oneself and one's family—distrust in family stories and local histories that have been passed down. Second, both women's narratives of historical trauma are intricately connected and remembered with and alongside contemporary forms of structural violence, symbolic violence, and everyday violence. Poverty, material dispossession, and poor health among family members and/or in themselves, as well as dependence on food and nutrition assistance, are products of historical, social, political, and economic forces that have displaced these women and constrained their capabilities and "freedom to achieve" (Sen 1988). "Home" for them is the impoverished and forgotten rural communities where life is lived at the edge of the world, and slow death (in the form of obesity and related illnesses) stunts future-bearing potentiality (Belcourt 2018).

Third, both women described feeling misery in the forms of anxiety, shame, or low self-esteem related to Indianness in multiple ways, and linked this misery with health outcomes.[30] For Linda, alcoholism—which she describes as hereditary for Indians and exacerbated by external factors and experiences—is a deep source of shame and destruction. For Sherry, racism and the positive association of Indianness *only* with social and financial benefits contributes to her shame and low self-esteem, a low self-esteem that she describes as *the* "Indian disease." For Linda and Sherry, their experiences of misery are directly related to health, and furthermore, this misery is part of what being Indian means, components of their Choctaw identity (or a broader Indian identity) pulled from a collective imagination that underpins local notions of Indianness. These are notions which present as real effects of social, political, and economic marginalization embodied within individuals, collectively affecting entire communities. Finally, obesity and diabetes affect both women's lives, placed not necessarily at the center of their stories but rather as intersecting conditions, symbiotic with other life experiences of being Indian. As Billy-Ray Belcourt (2018:2) describes it, "The feeling of indigeneity is the miserable feeling of not properly being of this world, and a disease like *Diabetes mellitus* is a key manifestation of this sort of exhausted existence. . . . Indigeneity is a zone of biological struggle." Combined, these key factors of historical trauma; structural, symbolic, and everyday violence; heritage; and identity make up the embodied heritage framework and contribute to how women make sense of their lived experiences of obesity and related conditions.

I position stories like Linda's and Sherry's in the larger political discourse that attributes a rise in obesity and diabetes among Native Americans to the links between health disparities (especially dependence on food and nutrition programs) and the dismantling of Indigenous cultures (Blackstock et al. 2006; Broussard et al. 1995; Candib 2007; Ferreira and Lang 2006; Roy 2006; Story et al. 1999). This is exemplified in both women's stories of poverty, growing up on commodities, and their dependence on food programs throughout their lives, providing the most acute illustration of how macro-level phenomena become realized in individual experience. During their lives, both women describe the foods they ate (e.g., white rice, bug-infested grains from the government, etc.) which informed their and their families' food and taste preferences into adulthood. Both Linda and Sherry could list and identify Choctaw foods, but neither knows how to cook them or recalled their own families cooking them much (or at all, in Linda's case). Their experiences as described, as well as the linkages between health, poverty, and cultural dismantling across women's stories, must be understood in the context of settler colonialism. As Patrick Wolfe (2006:388) notes, "Settler colonizers come to stay: invasion is a structure, not an event." Genocide is enacted alongside other measures, like erasure of foodways, with the goal of eliminating Indigenous peoples. This may occur violently (and indeed does), but elimination also occurs *following* efforts that aim to "produce life," such as assimilating Indigenous peoples, cultures, and lands into the body of the settler nation (Wolfe 1999, 2001). This process is precisely what narrows or erases possibilities of distinctive Indigenous nationalities challenging the goals and ambitions of the settler nation that is currently replacing them on their own lands.[31] Linda's and Sherry's descriptions of cultural knowledge—the ways traditional expressions of Choctaw culture have changed to become simultaneously more visible and unrecognizable—illustrate these efforts of erasure and replacement through the process of "producing life" within the settler nation. This violence cannot be separated from historical processes and is intricately tied to health and the ways that these women make sense of their current health experiences.

For Linda and Sherry, for Choctaws, and for many people all over the world, *commensality* (Counihan 2002) signifies intimacy, equality, and inclusion. Sherry called it "food and fellowship" and described the ways it brings people together. Alternatively, not eating together signifies distance, hierarchy, and social exclusion, and this was described in Linda's account of cooking eggs for her mother and the abuse that followed. Eating together forges social connections. And yet, across the project, Choctaw families rarely eat meals together at home and rarely invite guests into their homes to eat. Linda described cooking for herself and her grandson (when he is home), but they sit in front of the television to eat, or they eat at different times and different places in the house. Sherry described how her family had guests on Sundays when she was a child and how the guests got the best parts of the chicken, but she said she rarely has anyone over to her home to eat as an adult. Only in public places does food continue to unite Choctaws—for example, at church dinners, family reunions (most often held at churches), birthdays (usually held at restaurants), and fundraisers (held at various locations, including churches, community centers, schools, and CNO buildings). This leaves more questions than answers, but it can also be understood as part of the continued chipping away of Indigenous kinship that is inherent in settler colonialism and tied to a dependence on commodity foods.[32]

With the breakup of commensality in Choctaw families, as well as the dependence on commodity foods, foodways change, *food voice* (Hauck-Lawson 1998) wanes, and belief and family systems unravel. Food is imbued with social meaning, including its acquisition, preparation, provisioning, and cleanup. Hauck-Lawson's (1998) concept of *food voice* argues that what a person chooses to procure, prepare, and eat—and what a person does not choose—can make powerful statements about identity and culture. When foods and foodways change in a generation, as has occurred among Choctaws, and food choices become constrained by what the government selects for a group of people, the concept of the food voice is constrained as individual choice is constrained: Thus, food voice here additionally focuses on *when* Choctaws eat together. In the private sphere, women described their foodways from childhood to the present, and their food voice was quiet: They revealed dispossession, loss, and change. They had been dispossessed of their lands and food-related traditions; they lost their gardens, along with their knowledge of subsistence and traditional teachings; and they have "made do" with the rapid changes in foodways brought on by government-supplied foods. Yet, Choctaws' food voice is loud and clear when they gather together publicly to eat, to celebrate, and to be together, thus revealing the positions, values, and actions of Choctaws: "food and fellowship."

Conclusion

As this chapter demonstrates, food-centered life history narratives function as unique windows into the lives of individuals and their experiences with obesity and related conditions. In these two narratives, Linda and Sherry's stories reveal, for example, their health status, economic realities, psycho-emotional states, social networks, and family concerns. Food and foodways in these stories also reflect polytemporality: Food memories placed the women in the past and the present, and thus, created situations for recollections in the future, helping to shape a collective or social memory. (This is an important concept underpinning identity that I will return to in the next chapter.) Finally, their food-centered life history narratives situate their individual experiences within the larger constructs of historical trauma and contemporary violences, including poverty, oppression, dependency, and racism. Without narrative-level analysis, it would be easy to dismiss the women in this study as simply obese, or unhealthy, or poor, or victims. Yet, both immense suffering and incredible resilience seep through Linda's and Sherry's stories, and their narratives reveal *survivance* (Atalay 2006; Vizenor 1999). Their stories remind us to look beyond notions of victimhood and failure, to understanding the more complex narratives of Indian people and communities that neither ignore the larger settler-colonial context, nor focus only on the continued existence of Indians in the face of settler-colonialism.

Indeed, the stories show how important it is to understand the intersections of the structural, social, interpersonal, historical, and biological factors that contribute to the health and well-being of the women in the sample at large and the ways that they make sense of these experiences. In the next chapter, I present the major forms of historical and contemporary traumas (violences) described in the women's stories that give shape to the embodied heritage framework and demonstrate how these experiences—*and the ways that women make sense of them*—intersect and figure into obesity and cultural identity. The intersections of these multiple forces indicate the complexity of their experiences and that understanding such interconnection requires in-depth study and creative interventions that move beyond "quick fix" approaches. However, simply focusing on women's stories without moving to systematically evaluate all the different intersections remains limited too, in that it does not show specific ways in which narrative accounts might communicate actualized disease. Chapters 3, 4, and 5, therefore, move beyond narrative analysis at the textual level and use grounded theory to systematically catalogue the ways historical trauma, violence, heritage, identity, and obesity are reported across the project. Explained in depth, these themes set up a conceptual framework for a more detailed exploration of food, identity, and obesity.

CHAPTER 3

Historical Trauma, Contemporary Violence

Over the past four decades, theories of historical trauma have increasingly appeared across the literature in regard to individual and community health. *Historical trauma* refers to a complex, cumulative, and collective trauma experienced over time and across generations by a group of people who share an affiliation, circumstance, or identity (Brave Heart et al. 1995, 2011; Crawford 2014; Evans-Campbell 2008; Mohatt et al. 2014). Scholars from various disciplines have employed constructs of historical trauma to describe the impacts and legacies of colonization, cultural and material dispossession, and historical oppression (Braveheart et al. 1995; Evans-Campbell 2008; Gone 2013, 2014; Sotero 2006). This is especially true among Indigenous peoples and other ethnic minority populations that experience significant disparate health outcomes. Proponents of historical trauma frameworks have largely been mental and behavioral health professionals and advocates, and so the vast majority of historical trauma scholars call on established mental and behavioral health discourses with the goal of contextualizing, de-stigmatizing, and/or legitimizing Indigenous health problems, recovery, and cultural healing practices (Kirmayer et al. 2014).

The widespread interest in historical trauma has prompted a call for ways to make sense of the diverse empirical literature, particularly for ways to integrate the literature with theory to advance scientific inquiry

(Gone 2014; Mohatt et al. 2014). One such approach is the shift to understanding historical trauma as public narrative (Mohatt et al. 2014). That is, that a narrative approach, rather than an event-based understanding of historical trauma, may be more useful in connecting past historical injustices with contemporary experiences and circumstances of structural violence that influence health today (e.g., Crawford 2014; Kirmeyer et al. 2014; Mohatt et al. 2014). Indeed, framing historical trauma as a public narrative shifts the focus from searching for distal factors to explain contemporary health outcomes to one that examines how historical trauma is utilized in tribal communities (e.g., experienced as part of local and individual narratives of Indigenous health). Mohatt and colleagues (2014) offer a useful heuristic for how historical trauma as public narrative works: Contemporary narratives of historical wrongs are subject to present-day, public and personal *reminders* of historical trauma, and these in turn influence the degree to which historical trauma is salient and relevant for individuals. In other words, present-day experiences of injustice and disfranchisement are dialectically related to historical injustice and disfranchisement: Present experiences recall historical experiences, which in turn influence how (and to what degree) people link the present with the past. The embodied heritage framework utilizes Mohatt and colleagues' reframing of historical trauma as public narrative to understand the tangled and complex ways Choctaws link contemporary structural violence and inequities with past traumatic events.

This chapter begins with a brief review of historical trauma literature, including its origins and concepts, and introduces both the scholarly dialogue surrounding historical trauma and critiques of focusing on historical trauma as explanatory model for health outcomes, behaviors, and disease trends among Native Americans. Second, I examine the food-centered life history narratives to illustrate how experiences of historical trauma figure into women's meaning-making and to understand the role of historical trauma in the reporting of the narrative themes that emerged from them. Then, I present and unpack Nelly Coyote's story of historical trauma. Finally, I contend that historical trauma, and specifically the ways it is made sense of (i.e., historical trauma as public narrative), cannot be dissociated from contemporary structural violence, and further, together they are the root of poor health within this population.

Origins and Concepts

Historical trauma is defined as the "cumulative emotional and psychological wounding across generations, including the lifespan, which emanates from massive group trauma" (Brave Heart et al. 2011:283). Although multiple terms have been used to describe the intergenerational nature of distress,[1] *historical trauma* is the term used most often by scholars of Native American trauma (Evans-Campbell 2008).

The concept of *historical trauma* among Indigenous peoples first appeared in 1995 when Maria Yellow Horse Brave Heart applied theoretical contributions from Holocaust scholarship of collective suffering, unresolved grief, and trauma to the colonial conquest and federal assimilation policies experienced by the Lakota (Brave Heart and DeBruyn 1998). During her clinical training, Brave Heart, a Lakota social work researcher, recognized linkages between the genocide of European Jews during World War II and the Wounded Knee massacre of Lakotas in 1890 (Brave Heart and DeBruyn 1998; Gone 2014). Traumatic losses include forced removal and theft of land; violence and discrimination against Indigenous peoples; assimilation through residential schools and cultural suppression (i.e., language, ceremonies, and spirituality), as well as drastic changes to family systems and roles within families that led to cultural erosion and social destabilization (Brave Heart et al. 1998; Crawford 2014). Around the same time, Duran and Duran (1995) proposed the notion of the *soul wound* to characterize Indigenous suffering rooted in histories of colonial oppression, arguing that *soul wound* should be understood as historical context, rather than a construct, by service workers engaged with Indigenous peoples.[2] These early works by Indigenous scholars, originally located in mental health scholarship, aimed to historicize contemporary mental health disparities and substance abuse among Natives in light of past atrocities brought forth through colonization.

Historical trauma builds on theoretical and applied knowledge from the Holocaust survivor literature of the 1960s to argue for similar patterns of grief among Natives (Brave Heart 1995; Whitbeck et al. 2004).[3] In a series of seminal articles, Brave Heart (1998, 1999a, 1999b; Brave Heart and DeBruyn 1988, 1995) paralleled Native genocide, ethnic cleansing, and polices of forced assimilation with the Holocaust experience, noting similarities in the patterns of symptoms among Holocaust survivors and their families. Among Natives, she identified these as "symptoms of historical trauma" (Brave Heart 1998:288), and further refined the concept of *unresolved grief* to broadly apply to Indigenous peoples, describing historical trauma as "a deeper and more pervasive communal loss, resulting from genocide, massive human trauma over generations, [and] loss of land to which [Natives] were spiritually and emotionally tied" (Brave Heart and DeBruyn 1995:361).

In contrast to post-traumatic stress disorder (PTSD), historical trauma extends beyond the individual to include the family and community, as well as providing historical context to personal suffering. Gone (2014) notes that since these early introductions of historical trauma, scholars have elaborated and refined the construct as a distinctive explanatory model, or a set of beliefs, meanings, and expectations associated with a particular form of illness and its treatment (Kleinman et al. 1978). More recently, studies among other populations affected by violence and trauma have also documented the relationship between parental experiences of trauma and a historical trauma response among their children (Alexander 2004; Crawford 2014; Eyerman 2001; Rechtman 1997; Saito 2006; Sotero 2006; Zembylas and Bekerman 2008).[4] Furthermore, Whitbeck and colleagues (2004) developed the Historical Losses Scale (HLS) and the Historical Losses Associated Symptoms Scale, which aimed to generalize and measure historical trauma prevalence, its associated symptoms, and their severity. These scales have been used in larger studies among Natives with the goal of offering empirical evidence for historical trauma and, ultimately, legitimacy to its constructs.

However, historical trauma still lacks conceptual clarity. Brave Heart and colleagues (2011) state that the original intent of historical trauma was to frame current trauma exposure within the context of historical trauma to reduce stigma about emotional distress and responses to individual trauma and to highlight intergenerational collective trauma.[5] They distinguish between *historical trauma* and what they call the *historical trauma response* (Brave Heart et al. 2011). Again, *historical trauma* is defined as the "cumulative emotional and psychological wounding across generations, including the lifespan, which emanates from massive group trauma" (Brave Heart et al. 2011:283), whereas *historical trauma response* is defined as "a constellation of features associated with a reaction to massive group trauma" (Brave Heart et al. 2011:283). A component of the historical trauma response—unresolved grief—is noted as "the profound, unsettled bereavement resulting from cumulative devastating losses, compounded by the prohibition and interruption of Indigenous burial practices and ceremonies" (Brave Heart et al. 2011:283). Brave Heart and colleagues (2011) note that the intent of historical trauma and historical trauma response is to provide a context for the extreme emotional distress in Indigenous communities so as to ultimately foster healing.

Concepts of *historical trauma* were quickly picked up and circulated widely among Indigenous communities, as well as North American health service organizations and activists (e.g., Coyhis and Simonelli 2008; Prussing 2014; Wesley-Esquimaux and Smolewski 2004; Whitbeck et al. 2004). What seems to resonate particularly strongly is the conceptual model of historical trauma and historical trauma response linking experiences of lifetime traumatic events, as well as varying negative psychological outcomes for individuals, with often comorbid substance abuse.[6] But despite the increased interest in historical trauma as an explanation for current mental health disparities among Natives, there is relatively little empirical research documenting this phenomenon (Sotero 2006). This omission likely stems in part from the differing conceptualizations of historical trauma, but also because—despite Brave Heart and colleagues' (2011) attempts to distinguish between *historical trauma* and *historical trauma response*—the term *historical trauma* has been widely adopted as both a description of trauma responses and a causal explanation for them (Bombay et al. 2014; Evans-Campbell 2008; Walters et al. 2011).[7]

In perhaps the clearest (and most refined) contribution to historical trauma literature, Hartman and Gone (2014) identified four key components from the scholarship that characterize historical trauma. They refer to these four components as the "Four Cs of Indigenous Historical Trauma" (p. 275), and they include: 1) *Colonial injury* to Indigenous peoples as a consequence of experiences with conquest, subjugation, and dispossession by European and Euro-American settlers; 2) *Collective experience* of these injuries by entire Indigenous communities or collectivities whose identities, ideals, and social lives were impaired as a result; 3) *Cumulative effects* of these injuries from continued oppression that have accumulated over time through extended histories of harm by dominant settler-colonial society; and 4) *Cross-generational impacts* that result from these injuries as they are transmitted to subsequent generations in the form of legacies of risk and vulnerability to behavioral health problems until healing has occurred.

Historical trauma has been deployed by and within Indigenous communities to argue for addressing mental health disparities, namely by way of additional clinical interventions that focus on cultural revitalization (e.g., ceremonial participation) (Brave Heart and DeBruyn 1998; Gone and Trimble 2012), but also by situating historical trauma as a precipitating condition that influences health disparities (Sotero 2006; Walters and Simoni 2002; Williams et al. 2003). Robin and colleagues' (1996) research on PTSD argue that both specific and cumulative trauma among Natives are significant factors in high rates of substance abuse, traumatic depression, and PTSD. Walters and colleagues (2002) introduce an "Indigenist stress-coping model" that aims to understand vulnerabilities within the context of historic and contemporary oppression while also highlighting strengths and points of resiliency. Their approach positions Natives in a fourth-world context in which they live largely on the peripheries of a nation dominated by the colonizing majority with institutionalized power and privilege. Thus, Walters et al. (2002) regard contemporary stressors of poverty, racism, geography, and discrimination as part of the fourth-world dynamics that undermine the physical and mental health of Natives; they also note that historical and current traumas (e.g., unresolved grief and mourning related to loss of land and place; the negotiation of invisibility) affect Indigenous health. Yet, *how* it affects health has yet to be empirically documented.

In an attempt to delineate physical, psychological, and social pathways linking historical trauma to disease prevalence and health disparities, Sotero (2006) introduced a conceptual model whereby historical trauma originates with the subjugation by a dominant group, enforced in many ways, including military, bio-warfare, policies and/or laws of genocide, ethnic cleansing, prohibitions on economic development, and cultural expression.[8] The legacies of these overt and legitimized subjugations remain in the forms of racism, discrimination, and social and economic disadvantage, which constitute physical and psychological trauma for the affected population.[9] Sotero's conceptual model of historical trauma is an important contribution because it offers one of the first visual mappings of the "rich-in-variables framework" (2006:102) of historical trauma as a way forward in health disparities research. She contributes a detailed conceptual model that allows a dialectical relationship between the mental and physical effects of historical trauma. Equally important, her work recognizes the influence of contemporary experiences of social and structural vulnerability that may work as "triggers" linking the past (trauma) to the present (trauma).[10]

Critiques and Limitations

Several critiques have arisen surrounding theories of historical trauma. Scholars note the problematic nature of its origins in clinical mental health, namely the application of Western theories and methodologies to explain Indigenous peoples' experiences (Kirmayer et al. 2014; Maxwell 2014; McKinley 2012). In Kirmayer and colleagues' (2014) analysis of Native colonial distress and Jewish Holocaust distress, they contend that to compare the two, Indigenous historical trauma theory conflates historical events in ways that reduce suffering and distress to a uniform trans-historical/cultural phenomenon. Indeed, historical trauma argues that children of survivors in both communities share patterns of behavior and distress symptoms. Yet, often overlooked is that children of Holocaust survivors are generally doing better than their parents and grandparents across multiple measures (Kirmayer et al. 2014:311). This is not the case in many Indigenous communities, where rates of suicide, alcoholism, violence and abuse, and health inequities are much higher than national averages, and continue to increase in some communities. Thus, while historical trauma may play a causal role, we must also examine other, more proximate causal factors to account for the present distress and disparities in these populations.

McKinley (2012:141) argues that the pioneers of historical trauma theory have approached it with "Western tools as Indigenous discourse and then transferred to a Pan-Indian answer." Specifically, this means that historical trauma was conceived (and applied) in a clinical setting that essentially provided PTSD as a response to historically based collective traumas. Further, historical trauma is called upon to reflect an Indigenous world, ignoring culturally specific analyses and multi-cultural and

diverse settings (Gone and Kirmayer 2010). As such, this early and foundational work is circumscribed within a discourse of *pan-Indianism* yet
called *culturally specific*.[11]

A second set of critiques revolves around its pathways of transmission. First is the seemingly over-determined pathways of intergenerational transmission of historical trauma. Scholars note the means of such
transmissions are varied and include altered parenting, "cycle of abuse"
theories, distressing oral histories, and more recently, epigenetics. Yet,
the rush to explain the pathways of transmission often overlooks the
complexity of potential pathways and the fact that they may occur at
many levels. This includes interpersonally; within families; and at the
community, national, and international levels (UN General Assembly
2007). Maxwell (2014) problematizes the intergenerational transmission of historical trauma, situating its discourses as the "offspring" of
Native healing and colonial professional critiques of Indigenous family
life. She highlights the antithetical nature of the two: Native healing is
concerned with a therapeutic approach to restoring intergenerational
social relations, while the other has pathologized Indigenous parenting
and child-rearing practices.[12] Her main critique is with the pathway of
intergenerational transmission of historical trauma via parenting, arguing that it works to (re)blame parents and grandparents by pathologizing Indigenous families. This further promotes an oversimplified,
universalizing understanding of colonization in which Indigenous peoples are *always and only* victims, thus diverting attention from the contemporary continuation of colonial institutions, structures, discourses,
practices, and relations that disrupt Indigenous family life in the present
(Maxwell 2014).

More recently, scholars have identified epigenetic processes at the biological level of transmission. That is, "At the cellular level . . . powerful
stressful environmental conditions can leave an imprint or 'mark' on the
epigenome (cellular genetic material) that can be carried into future generations with devastating consequences" (Walters et al. 2011:11). However, Kirmayer and colleagues (2014) warn that this trend may translate
to "fashionable forms of biological reductionism [that] may not serve
the emancipatory goals of Indigenous decolonization . . . [and] there
is no reason to assume that epigenetic mechanisms—which appear to
be reversible with appropriate life experiences—would not operate in

service to intergenerational resilience as much as to intergenerational trauma" (2014:309). Hence, any analysis of the transmission of historical trauma across generations must recognize that although there may be complex interactions across levels, each level involves multiple and unique processes which are irreducible to the lower levels. While "postulated biological mechanisms" may seem to provide a more fundamental level of analysis (and understanding), privileging one level of explanation over another will lead to an incomplete understanding and may prevent a deeper understanding of processes at other levels (Kirmayer et al. 2014:310).

Additionally, establishing definite causal linkages across generations is perhaps impossible because retrospective studies are constrained by limited data and recall bias (Kirmayer et al. 2014; Mohatt et al. 2014). Kirmayer and colleagues (2014:307) argue that simply because people attribute their problems to past traumatic events, this does not prove a causal link, and more importantly, it may be the result of a "looping effect." That is, the more popular the concept of historical trauma becomes, the more likely people are to frame their problems and think about their experiences in ways that line up with the model. A perverse outcome, they argue, is that Indigenous cultural identity then comes to signify ancestral victimization in a way that necessarily adopts "a narrow and overgeneralized form of historical consciousness" expressed and endorsed by psychological distress (Kirmayer et al. 2014:307).[13]

Furthermore, the concept of historical trauma links the persistent suffering of Indigenous peoples in the past, redirecting an examination of ongoing structural violence in the present that contributes to inequities among Indigenous peoples today. Maxwell's (2014) critique draws attention to how historical trauma theory has retooled the parameters of discussions of particular trauma experiences (e.g., boarding schools), raising questions about the broader implications of the contemporary political, social, and moral contexts in which "experiences of abuse carry proportionately greater currency than collective experiences of structural violence" (Maxwell 2014:419). Furthermore, she argues that the framework of historical trauma, then, is seen in a way that fosters the remembering and wide circulation of *certain* histories while, at the same time, facilitates the marginalization and forgetting of other histories, thus distracting attention from the present inequities.

Dian Million's (2013) critique of trauma discourse underscores how colonial violence and Indigenous dispossession are often reframed as individual psychological suffering rather than recognized as ongoing structural injustices. While trauma studies and healing narratives have helped Indigenous communities articulate harm and reclaim their voices, Million warns that these frameworks often serve state interests rather than advancing Indigenous sovereignty. She argues that trauma discourse pathologizes Indigenous women specifically, reducing their experiences to interpersonal violence while obscuring settler colonialism's role in producing systemic harm. This medicalization shifts responsibility onto individuals for their own healing, frequently through biomedical therapeutic models, rather than addressing the broader political-economic conditions that sustain Indigenous suffering. Million's concept of therapeutic nations critiques how the state manages Indigenous trauma through institutionalized healing programs that emphasize resilience and self-transformation, reinforcing neoliberal governance rather than collective resistance. Governments and non-profits, she argues, acknowledge Indigenous suffering through trauma discourse but fail to address its root causes—such as land dispossession, economic marginalization, and systemic inequities—offering symbolic recognition without material redistribution.

Gone (2014) extends Million's critique by questioning how historical trauma functions as a "powerful moral rhetoric" that implicates European and Euro-American colonization in pervasive Indigenous psychosocial problems. While he acknowledges its political and discursive potency, he warns against its essentialist implications, particularly the assumption that all Indigenous peoples are universally wounded by history. Gone challenges the idea that Indigenous experiences of colonization were monolithic, arguing instead for attention to the diverse ways communities have responded, resisted, and adapted. Like Million, he critiques the tendency to focus on historical trauma in ways that emphasize past harm while neglecting the ongoing structural inequalities that actively disadvantage Indigenous peoples today. He also cautions against historical trauma becoming a polarizing construct that simplifies race relations into a binary of oppressed and oppressor, arguing that future generations must engage with these issues in ways that move beyond merely condemning colonial history to instead securing justice in the present.

While Million (2013) and Gone (2014) both critique trauma discourse for its potential to depoliticize and essentialize Indigenous experiences, Million foregrounds the ways neoliberal governance co-opts trauma as a tool of state control, while Gone warns against using historical trauma as a reductive framework that risks overlooking contemporary struggles and diversities within Indigenous communities. Million, however, also recognizes the power of Indigenous storytelling as a political tool that resists colonial erasure. While such narratives can serve as acts of defiance and reclamation, she warns that institutions may appropriate them in ways that depoliticize their radical potential. Ultimately, both scholars call for a rethinking of Indigenous healing that moves beyond state-sanctioned therapeutic recognition to focus on sovereignty, land reclamation, and structural justice.

A clear thread throughout these critiques points toward the positioning of historical trauma theory: It is situated largely within an essentialist framework (e.g., of binary oppositions) and, equally importantly, has missed the importance of meaning-making. These are critical and under-explored problems with the body of knowledge surrounding historical trauma. Specifically, there is at once an oppositional, reductionistic, essentializing thinking underlying historical trauma theory that directs the discourse and perpetuates oppositions[14] while also missing the important ways that historical trauma as a framework is "put to work" or utilized among Indigenous individuals and communities to make sense of contemporary experiences of inequities. While critics of historical trauma theory acknowledge both its reliance on essentialized categories and its practical use within Indigenous communities, these aspects remain largely unexamined and insufficiently theorized. Moreover, positional binaries and limited understanding of historical trauma as praxis leave very limited space for alternative ways of thinking (e.g., fluidity, back and forth), ways of experiencing (e.g., contemporary structural violence), and ways of making sense of the world.

Additionally, the location of much of the current historical trauma theory within the fields of mental and behavioral health has meant that its relevance to the conditions of everyday life in the present is often oblique. In fact, there is wide agreement that the constructs of historical trauma are useful in implicating colonization in the onset and maintenance of pervasive and ongoing health and social problems among Indigenous peoples. Historical trauma offers a framing that community members, grassroots advocates, healthcare and services providers, educators, researchers, and other professionals can (and do) get behind when advocating for Indigenous health equities. Although the pathways or mechanisms of how it actually functions are not entirely clear or agreed upon—and the diversity of politics found among its many supporters, coupled with its conceptual murkiness, makes things messy—the historical trauma "movement" (although flawed in many ways) resonates with Indigenous people, families, and communities. In other words, historical trauma theory is being utilized in ways that reflect how people complexly understand, make sense of, and apply notions of historical trauma in their everyday lives.

The next section of this chapter explores how and in what ways historical trauma theory is "put to work" in a local context, specifically in themes that have emerged from the food-centered life history interviews, as well as the ways in which historical trauma is used to make sense of everyday life in the Choctaw Nation. This is a crucial piece of the embodied heritage framework.

Historical Losses and Women's Stories

Recall Linda's and Sherry's stories from chapter 2; historical trauma was prevalent in both their narratives. For Linda, alcoholism was identified as a major byproduct of trauma, with drinking and diabetes synonymous with Indian identity. She admitted to drinking throughout her pregnancies, drinking to cope with her divorce, and drinking as a way to pass time with her relatives. She also identified the multiple forms of abuse her mother had inflicted upon her and linked this abuse with her mother's "hard life," alluding to boarding schools. However, Linda didn't know much about her mother's boarding school experiences; in fact, Linda expressed not knowing much about her parents at all. Indeed, this is one of the most prevalent forms of historical trauma I uncovered among women in this research (through their interviews): the unsaid; the unknown; the loss, disruption, and interruption; all creating pain and sadness, often numbed, silenced, or exacerbated with alcohol, abuse, shame, and stigma.

For Sherry, historical trauma is used to make sense of the ways in which stigma and shame occupy much of what it means to be Indigenous for her generation. She described her experiences of racism at church, her brother's white wife encouraging him to identify as Choctaw only for "benefits," and the loss of traditions and respect for elders, linked with ruptures in cultural knowledge and transmission. Throughout the food-centered life history interviews, women continuously brought up historical trauma in their narratives, using it as a construct to make sense of their food and foodways experiences, their identities and heritage, and even their parenting experiences, including breastfeeding. For many, historical trauma was indirectly or passingly implicated, and for others, it was directly linked and called upon as explanation for their experiences. Importantly, however, historical trauma was consistently linked with contemporary experiences. That is, it was used as a public narrative (Mohatt et al. 2014) to make sense of or to explain contemporary experiences of structural violence.

I next present findings from the Historical Losses Scale (HLS) to systematically examine the frequency with which Choctaws in this research think about losses associated with historical trauma; then I offer findings from the food-centered life history interviews around the most prevalent losses to better understand the experiences of historical trauma in this sample.

Historical Losses Scale (HLS)

Historical losses were reported to be much on the minds of the women in this study, many of whom are, themselves, part of the Indian boarding school and relocation era—either having been sent to boarding school or having a relative (e.g., parent, grandparent, aunt, uncle, etc.) who was sent to Indian boarding schools. Thus, they are not necessarily several generations past the worst atrocities of assimilation policies. Nearly one-third of the women reported thinking monthly or more often (i.e., weekly, daily, several times a day) regarding loss of land; more than half (56 percent) of women had such thoughts yearly or during special times and occasions. More than a quarter of the women (28 percent) thought at least weekly about loss of Choctaw language and religion/spirituality (27 percent). This increased to almost half of all participants when those who had such thoughts at least monthly were taken into consideration. Much fewer reported recurrent thoughts of loss of family ties because of boarding schools or relocation (8 percent at least weekly for both); only when the specified timeframe was yearly or at special times did this statistic increase (52 percent and 71 percent, respectively). Poor treatment by government officials was more recurrent, with 15 percent thinking of this weekly or more (and an additional 15 percent thinking of this monthly). Almost one-fourth thought monthly or more about broken treaties, and this increased to two-thirds when those who thought of broken treaties yearly or at special times were included. A quarter of women thought weekly or more about losing their culture; this increased dramatically when a rate of yearly or more was included (86 percent). Alcoholism was very much on everyone's mind. Only 4 percent "never" thought of it. Almost a quarter of women thought of it daily or more, and almost 35 percent thought of alcoholism at least weekly. Loss of respect for elders was the most recurring and the most lamented theme, with nearly 30 percent thinking of this daily or more (this increased to 61 percent when those who thought of it at least monthly were considered). Loss because of early deaths was thought of at least weekly by more than one-quarter of participants, and at least monthly by more than half of them. Finally, loss of respect by children for traditional ways was thought of daily or more by 22 percent of the women, and monthly or more by almost half of them.

These frequencies indicate that the women in this study are very much in touch with the historical losses of their people. In fact, nearly 40 percent of the women thought monthly or more about historical losses. But while the Historical Losses Scale (HLS) is useful in assessing the frequency of specific losses associated with historical trauma, the ways in which the women spoke about their losses is much more telling. First, "yearly or special times" is the most frequently reported timeframe across items, yet to assume that "special times" is equivalent with "yearly" (as is implied by their being lumped together in the HLS) would be inaccurate in this sample. Women's stories, as well as the ethnography of this research, show that "special times" include those times when families get together and tell stories. This happens more frequently than yearly—as often as monthly—because, in addition to family reunions, "special times" include birthdays, graduation parties, funerals, and other

TABLE 2 Summary of participants' responses on the historical losses scale

Items (Loss of . . .)	Never	Yearly or Special Times	Monthly	Weekly	Daily	Several Times a Day
Land	8.3%	56.3%	14.6%	8.3%	4.2%	2.1%
Language	4.3%	40.4%	19.1%	12.8%	8.5%	6.4%
Traditional spiritual ways	6.3%	39.6%	16.7%	10.4%	12.5%	4.2%
Family ties, due to boarding schools	39.6%	43.8%	0%	4.2%	0%	4.2%
Families, due to relocation	16.7%	54.1%	8.3%	6.3%	2.1%	0%
Self-respect, due to poor treatment by government officials	25%	35.4%	14.6%	4.2%	8.3%	2.1%
Trust in whites, due to broken treaties	20.8%	43.8%	12.5%	4.2%	6.3%	0%
Culture	4.2%	41.7%	18.8%	10.4%	8.3%	6.3%
Miscellaneous, due to effects of alcoholism on our people	4.3%	28.3%	21.7%	13%	15.2%	6.5%
Respect by our children and grandchildren for their elders	10.9%	21.7%	19.6%	13%	19.6%	8.7%
People due to early deaths	6.5%	34.8%	23.9%	10.9%	17.4%	0%
Respect by our children for our traditional ways	8.7%	37%	15.2%	8.7%	17.4%	4.3%

Note: Percentages (%) are rounded and do not include "Don't Know" responses; therefore, % will not add up to 100%.

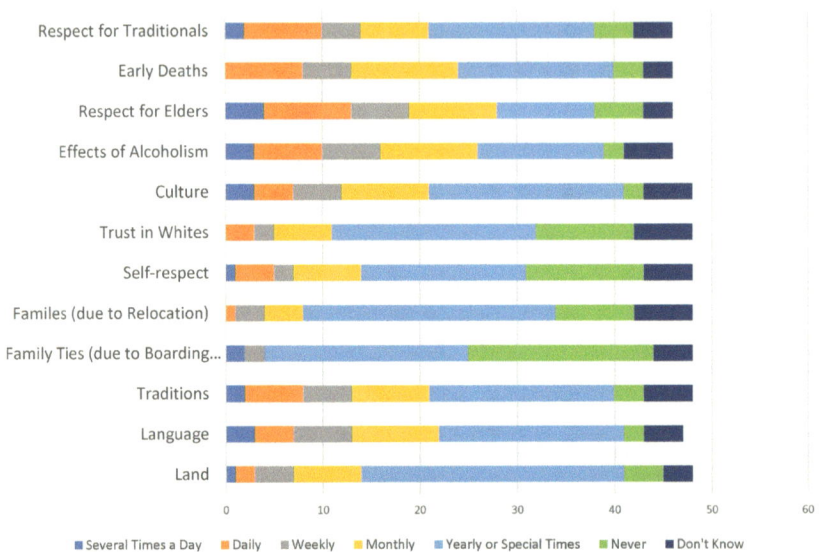

FIGURE 8 Historical losses scale. Graph by Kasey Jernigan (author).

celebrations or remembrances. In large families, these types of "special times" can, and do, occur frequently. Additionally, many of the women spoke about these losses as clusters, so they identified loss of language as not separate from loss of land, for example. Therefore, I explore these themes interconnectedly, as they were shared with me.

The majority of Choctaws do not speak *Chahta anumpa* (the Choctaw language), and UNESCO[15] has designated it as endangered (level 1, vulnerable). The Choctaw Nation has widely implemented community language courses, available for free at all the community centers, online, in select local high schools as a foreign language option,[16] and in collaboration with colleges and universities across the state. Several women described a sort of interstitial experience now that the Nation is (re) teaching *Chahta anumpa*: Many of their elders can speak *Chahta*, and their children are learning and speaking it, so the women interviewed in this research identify as in-between generations and often feel lost or left out. Often, they find themselves learning from their children (or even grandchildren) how to pronounce a word or to say something in *Chahta*, thus destabilizing their roles as elders and knowledge holders.

Yet, they are fully aware of and reiterate the very reasons for why they cannot speak *Chahta*; they recall boarding school experiences and the U.S. government's determination to erase *Chahta anumpa*. In other words, historical trauma is called upon to explain both why they cannot speak *Chahta* as well as a way to maintain their in-group status (i.e., *not* knowing *Chahta anumpa* is a specific experience that informs what it means to be Choctaw for this generation).

> My kids didn't learn [*Chahta anumpa*] from me or my husband. But we have their grandparents, my mother and my in-laws, they are fluent speakers. So my son, he went to work for [the language department] several years ago, so he was around it, and he had a strong desire to learn. He was around it so much, he just started picking up on it. So, he can conversate now. He understands a lot. Like when he comes back, he'll conversate with his aunts, grand aunts, his grandparents, and so they'll just be rambling on and on. When they're talking and stuff, and sometimes they'll say something, I'll say, "I know you're talking about me . . . I don't know exactly what you're saying, but I know you said—whatever, I know you said something." When he started, then I felt bad because I thought, "Oh, gosh, I didn't learn it." But it wasn't no fault of ours. And I understand why my parents and my grandparents didn't fully implement that in their children. I understand that, but now, it's like we're going backwards and trying to learn it. (Carmen, Broken Bow)

> But growing up my mom was fluent, my dad was fluent, my grandpa, my biological grandma was fluent too, but I never knew her but my step-grandmother was fluent. In the church, people were fluent so you pick up things. My mom didn't want us speaking Choctaw because she said it's a white man's world and you have to speak English. My oldest sister, she does, and my oldest brother, and they're about the only two that can carry on a conversation with you. The rest of us, you know, my dad would [be] at the table, and he would always say, "Pass the bread," in Choctaw or, you know, "Give it to me." If I got it and gave it to him, he'd laugh at me [laughter]. He didn't know if I knew what he was talking about. He'd chuckle, "Ah ha ha ha ha," [laughter] because he didn't think that I would know what he's talking about." (Billie, Durant)

Well, I think it is a good idea [that the Nation is teaching *Chahta*] because none of us know how to speak. See, my granddaughter, she can understand it, she can speak most of it, she can sing it. I can't do any of that. She came back here and started taking some [*Chahta*] in school, so she can do that, and I can't. And, I have to ask her sometimes what this word is, or how do you pronounce it, or translate however you want to say—that is why I have to ask her. (Mandy, Broken Bow)

Like Linda, numerous participants expressed a profound lack of knowledge regarding their familial histories. They were unaware of the circumstances that led their families to settle in these specific small towns, the origins of their parents' relationships, reasons behind relocations, or even basic family lineage details. For those with some knowledge, there existed a pervasive distrust of the information they possessed, primarily because it demanded they hold conflicting narratives. For example, the dominant narratives taught in educational settings in Oklahoma and across the United States teach that the land was unassigned, free, and available for settlement, whereas Choctaw narratives recall the many ways land was stolen. This dichotomy fostered uncertainty and ambivalence within personal narratives, their onto-epistemologies eroded by time, institutionalized narratives, and the impact of structural violence.

Women articulated complex insights into historical trauma, making connections between past losses and their current realities as Choctaw women. They invoked it as a framework for understanding the interplay between historical events and contemporary experiences. For instance, they associated the historical dispossession of land with the procurement of commodities and, consequentially, the rise of diabetes among Natives in general. They further linked mental illness and substance abuse to historical trauma, recognizing alcohol abuse in particular as a form of self-medication. They also implicated alcohol historically in unfair land exchanges and dispossession of all sorts, contributing to a legacy of alcohol use in their communities. Although commodities now include beneficial items like fresh fruits and vegetables, the prevalence of sugars and salts are linked in their stories to widespread diabetes and viewed as a prolongation of the historical poisoning of Natives. These narratives underscore the enduring impact of historical trauma on health and social dynamics within Indigenous communities. That is, they frequently connected historical losses with their contemporary experiences, calling on historical trauma as public narrative to make sense of their lives as Choctaws today.

The *language* of historical trauma was not used among the participants, although most women had engaged in discussions implicating it—both with their families and within Indian communities—without explicitly naming it as such. An illustrative example is provided by Nelly Coyote, whose narrative is detailed later in this chapter. Familiar with literature on the Holocaust and associated trauma research, Nelly made intuitive connections between the genocide of Native Americans and related trauma despite being unaware of existing historical trauma research specific to Indigenous communities. Importantly, these women's discussions about historical trauma and losses diverged from abstract historical discourse; instead, they addressed trauma and loss as impacting family members in the present day. When Nelly Coyote recounted her mother's profound emotional reaction whenever discussing the Trail of Tears, how her mother appeared to be in physical pain, it led her to believe, as a child, that her mother had personally walked the Trail of Tears. This anecdote highlights how, for these women, the temporal distance to such traumatic events is perceived differently. Their vivid and empathetic narration ensures that history's painful losses remain palpably present in their bodies, their stories, and the broader collective narrative.

Another illustrative case of historical trauma and associated losses, not accounted for by the Historical Loss Scale (HLS), is the disruption of traditional roles of women as teachers and knowledge holders, particularly in the context of breastfeeding practices. Breastfeeding offers numerous health benefits, including reducing the risk of diabetes and obesity, and breastmilk is the most important first food in a baby's life. However, data from 2016 report that in the CNO region, 83 percent of infants were formula-fed, and only 12 percent of infants were exclusively breastfed, meaning they consumed only breastmilk and no formula (USDA/FNS Supplemental Food Programs Division 2017). Indeed, very few of the women in this project had had the experience of breastfeeding their children or being breastfed themselves. Compounding this issue was their present inability to provide guidance on breastfeeding to their own daughters. They traced this back to when, as young mothers themselves, (non-Native) medical professionals at Indian hospitals explicitly discouraged them from breastfeeding, claiming, for example, that their breastmilk was "spoiled," "not pure," or "weak," or claiming the baby was "lactose intolerant."[17] Consequently, these women did not breastfeed and later lacked the capacity to instruct their own daughters and granddaughters, yet again troubling their roles as elders and knowledge holders. Additional reasons for not breastfeeding included feeling embarrassed to breastfeed in public—and especially being discouraged by men for seemingly "exposing" themselves—but also, some had a baby born with a tooth or just didn't like how it felt to breastfeed. Notably, many of these women had babies when they were still teenagers and, in hindsight, said they were also so young and unknowledgeable about the benefits of breastfeeding. These narratives underscore the ways in which external influences, and particularly discrimination, including narratives about "dirty Indians," have destabilized and disrupted the intergenerational transmission of breastfeeding knowledge and practices, highlighting yet another broader impact of historical trauma on Indigenous communities.

Finally, before presenting Nelly Coyote's story, I introduce another woman, Sammy: She is a fifty-three-year-old Muscogee Creek woman who lives with her Choctaw partner on the Choctaw reservation. Sammy contacts me after seeing my recruitment flyer at one of the commodity foods distribution stores. She has been eager to talk with me, she tells me, and has hitched a ride with the tribal transportation service to the hospital (because the van is available only for medical appointments and commodity food pick up). From there, she has walked the remaining two miles to the public library where we meet.

Sweaty and out of breath, Sammy has barely sat down before beginning in a rapid, matter of fact tone:

> I do get commodities, and for the most part they're really good, but in a lot of ways, they're just continuing to poison [us] like they have been doing for hundreds of years now as far as I'm concerned. We do get some really good things, some fresh fruits and vegetables now that we didn't used to. We get good meat, but the other things . . . So many of us are diabetic, obese, sick.

Sammy pauses here, looks up at the ceiling, and continues:

You know that saying, "You don't know what you don't know"? Well, we know what we don't know. . . . It's been a very long process of alienating us from our culture. Back when the Dawes Rolls came about, there were so many Indians that would not sign on the Dawes Roll, that's why some of us are, I guess, fortunate enough to be, as my daddy called it, "card-carrying Indians." But there is a lot of them, a lot of Indians here, their ancestors would sign the Rolls, and one of the many reasons was, the deal was: "You sign here, we give you some of the land that used to belong to you to start with, but you got to break up your tribal ways. . . . You can't live in the tribal community anymore. You have to split up in separate households and live like white people do." And when you strip those kinds of things away from people . . . when you start separating us . . .

Sammy sighs deeply here, then continues:

And now here we are, out in these places [reservations], out in the middle of nowhere, with insufficient housing, insufficient water, insufficient sewage, insufficient food—not that we don't get enough food, but the kind of food we're given to make do with is completely against hell. When all these things happen, people don't know how to be who they're supposed to be—we don't know the stories we're supposed to know, we don't have the traditional teachings we're supposed to have, and then we begin to lose respect for ourselves. There doesn't seem to be any point in much of anything else. It's like the white man said, "You're an Indian but you can't do this, and you can't be this, and you can't speak that . . ." So many of us are diabetic—almost every Native I know is diabetic. High blood pressure, obesity, alcoholism, all brought on by loss of our culture. . . . I see in myself some of my dad's ways. He used to call it, you just "go Indian." You just shut down. Quiet. Just "go Indian."

Tears roll down Sammy's cheeks; she lets them fall, refusing to wipe them away.

Sammy's narrative offers a compelling exploration of historical trauma through a personalized lens and, especially, interweaves past and present. She navigates temporality, tying historical acts of violence to modern structural injustices. Such articulation was intentional among the women discussing historical trauma, offering a way to contextualize and make sense of their current experiences with structural violence. For Sammy, historical events provide a narrative context in which she interprets and makes sense of contemporary social issues, including health, identity (i.e., who counts as Indian and how that came to be), dismantling of Indigenous cultures, stereotypes of Indians, loss of self-worth, and alcoholism. Sammy draws on both personal experiences and broader collective narratives and histories, such as those related to life on reservations in general (not just the Choctaw Nation), which provide interpretative frameworks for her present-day experiences of violence. In this sense, it is Sammy's present conditions and experiences that make historical trauma relevant to the present and the future (Mohatt et al. 2014). Historical trauma narratives are highly salient and accessible to Sammy, and therefore current experiences of violence become readily apparent as part of the historical trauma narrative (Mohatt et al. 2014).

Next, I present Nelly Coyote's story and the ways in which daily indignities are embedded in narratives of historical trauma, thus serving as reminders and continuations of past trauma but also the ways in which historical trauma narratives work as narratives of ongoing resistance. The following story serves as a powerful example of how historical trauma narratives can simultaneously manifest a sense of loss and resilience.

Nelly Coyote's Story

Nelly Coyote,[18] a sixty-six-year-old Choctaw woman, is diabetic, clinically labeled as morbidly obese, and restricted to a wheelchair. She saw my recruitment flyer in the tribal newspaper, called me, and invited me to come to her home to conduct the interview. Her house, located in a tiny, rural town in the center of the Choctaw Nation, is a small, neat home with few furnishings. To accommodate her extra-wide wheelchair, her daughter has made multiple informal modifications throughout the house: She has hacked off the bottom halves of the trims around all the door frames, leaving them chipped, splintered, and unpainted. She has also ripped up the carpet, revealing exposed, unfinished subfloor so Nelly's wheelchair can move unrestricted. Nelly welcomes me inside her home, turns on the air conditioner in the kitchen, and serves me homemade iced tea and boiled peanuts as she begins to tell me her story.

Nelly Coyote has one daughter, Liza, and an adopted granddaughter, River. River is currently living with Nelly while Liza is in the Pacific Northwest visiting a friend and looking for work. Nelly Coyote's husband died several years ago and left behind a half-finished house next door that he had been building. When home, Liza spends her time working on the house, laying sheetrock and learning construction.

Nelly Coyote has moved around all her life, relocating every few years, because her father was a preacher.[19] She lived in dozens of small towns scattered across Oklahoma and Texas, spending the longest time (seven years) in Brownsville, Texas, but she calls Durant, Oklahoma, her original home because it is where her maternal grandparents lived. During high school, Nelly Coyote left home and moved to New York City, got a job at a Howard Johnson hotel chain, rented a hotel room near Times Square, and eventually enrolled in night school to get her GED. She spent most of her time in and out of relationships with different men, living and traveling the world with them.[20] After ten years in New York, Nelly Coyote moved back to Durant to take care of her ageing mother, but she could not find work and grew bored. She joined the military because she "couldn't get away again. It was too hard, and I didn't have any money, so I joined the Navy." Nelly Coyote's young adult life resembled her constantly changing childhood, and she relocated multiple times after the Navy, living in Austin, Los Angeles, Tulsa, and so on. In Los Angeles, she enrolled in the University of California Los Angeles (UCLA) and was majoring in philosophy; then her brother committed suicide. At that point, she left UCLA, moved back to Durant, and stayed in Oklahoma for good.

Both of Nelly's parents attended Indian boarding schools, snatched from their families as young children and sent hundreds of miles away for education. As teens, they both attended Chilocco Indian Agricultural High School, where they met and married shortly after graduating. Nelly tells me that because she was a philosophy major, she has spent a great deal of time reflecting on her family's narrative as a way to make sense of her own life (and her daughter's and granddaughter's lives). Additionally, her mother wrote a great deal—poems, stories, accounts, letters, etc.—and saved photos of her childhood, all of which Nelly has curated into a thick scrapbook serving as material culture of her family's histories. Commenting about her parent's boarding school experiences, Nelly Coyote shares:

They didn't have a perspective that I have now. They were taught that what they were taught was right. You know, their being there [at the boarding school] was right. It was a privilege, and they were taught the value of education.[21] They were educated. They went to college, both my parents, and got masters [degrees]. They believed in education, but they didn't know the ropes at all. They didn't know how to—but they still went through all the motions [*sighs deeply*]. I can see now, like, its purpose, but they didn't see it then.[22] And do you know what I noticed? The generation that went to Chilocco, they grew up there. They seem to be very together people. Like, they have jobs, they dress well. My aunts, they lived in nice houses . . . they all married people from Chilocco, they lived in [cities]. But this generation's children—us—we're a mess, a real mess! My older brother killed himself. My younger brother died when he was forty-one from chickenpox, but he was such a mess, it was a relief [when he died]. He was a mess!

Nelly continues to account for more family members—siblings, cousins, aunts, and so on—describing the many ways they have suffered from mental health issues, chronic illnesses, violence and homicide, cousins gone missing, and what she calls "social deviance."

Let's see, the only kind of normal, the people that knew the ropes a little bit, was the youngest girl's children. She's the aunt that's still alive—she didn't go to Chilocco . . . but she has children who . . . are kind of like what society expects you to be. The others, no it didn't happen that way . . . I read a book once . . . about children who were born after the Holocaust, but to parents who had been in the Holocaust. It rang true. It's like our family. . . . These [children who went to the boarding schools] were children taken away from their families and raised very regimentally. They had to march all the time and obey.

Her voice cracks, and she begins to cry but continues:

My family, when they talk to each other, they—I'm talking about that generation—they're very quiet. They tell each other all jokes, but they never let on. It's a secret way of being. I think that's the result of the boarding school. . . . They never were alright. My mother was never alright. . . . My father was completely crazy. . . . I lived with one aunt, [my father's] sister and her husband. They both went to Chilocco too, and my cousins—I lived with them for a few summers, and they weren't alright either. All kind of under-currents that you didn't know, you didn't understand at all.

Nelly Coyote stops here, sobbing, and pulls out tissues to wipe away the tears that have been streaming down her face. She brings out the book of her mother's writings and shows me as she continues talking.

Even the Trail of Tears, which I'm sure my mother only heard about or from reading—it wasn't being taught in history class or something. When she would tell me the story, she would cry. When I was growing up, I thought she had gone over the Trail of Tears. I didn't realize that she's talking about history. Anyway, that was my mother. That's her little book, her poems, and about her life, and her things.

Nelly Coyote's story is very painful for her to tell. She stops several times to collect herself and wipe away tears, and I think at first this is why her story feels scattered or all over the place. After our interview, I return to her story several times, reading the transcription and listening to her recorded voice, and it becomes clearer to me that she is surrounded by structural and physical contexts that remind her daily of the historical processes of loss, marginalization, discrimination, and trauma: the physical book of her mother's stories and poems about boarding schools; the loss and deaths of multiple family members; living in the small town she never wanted to return to; struggling with obesity and diabetes and no longer feeling beautiful; even the sawed off door frames and bare subfloors in her home are not simply adjustments for her oversized wheelchair but also represent decay, haunting her with memories of the past and particularly with possibilities that were only available in the past.[23] Nelly specifically links her family's multiple deaths and cultural dismantling with the boarding schools, and furthermore, these past traumas serve as the background story for her daughter, Liza, as well as her adopted granddaughter, River.

When Liza was in the eighth grade, Nelly Coyote sent her to Red River Preparatory School (RRPS), an elite private school in the city (160 miles away), after realizing that the schools in her town were not adequate for her daughter.[24] They secured financial aid at RRPS, rented a one-room apartment nearby the school, and Nelly Coyote got a part-time, minimum-wage job as a receptionist at a grief counseling center in the city so she could be present for Liza after school. For five years, they lived in the city during the school year, returning to their rural town for summers. While in the city, they depended on food banks because the commodities food program does not extend into the cities. Liza graduated from RRPS with honors and received a scholarship to attend a private liberal arts college in the Pacific Northwest, where she excelled: She majored in international political economy, studied abroad in Central and West Africa, and is fluent in four languages.

After graduating college, Liza returned home to their rural town to be with her mother, but according to Nelly Coyote, Liza cannot find employment, has difficulty with relationships and friendships, and is counting down the days until her college student loans are considered paid and she is no longer in debt. Nelly tells me about Liza:

> Liza is in [the Pacific Northwest] now. She went out there to school, and she has a friend from college there. She wanted to get away from this area, because it's—she doesn't meet other people her age who are educated. She doesn't have a boyfriend, and she doesn't . . . she has friends, but they're not on her par in some ways. She wanted a break, and she planned it. She is staying with her friend that she met in college and she's going to look for a job, part-time job. Two part-time jobs or something. She wants to be freer and have more money and make more friends. Eat better food. But she loves her home. . . . She was going to school here [in town]. See, she came home from school, that little school at the end of the road, and told me one day she is the smartest one in school, even smarter than her teachers, and I thought to myself that she probably was. And I had a friend who'd had a son in RRPS, that school in [the city]. I didn't realize what it was going to be like. I thought I was seeking a more intellectual school. I wanted her to have—you see, I went to college, and I've educated myself because I read a lot, and I just wanted her to be in an environment where she wasn't the smartest person so she could learn things, where she could learn languages and things like that. For instance, in one of the schools over here, the teacher said, "Well, if you're so smart, why don't you read this?" and handed her Shakespeare, in a put-down kind of way, and so of course she tried but couldn't make heads or tails out of it. But at RRPS,

they taught her how to read Shakespeare, and she learned! And that is what I was seeking. I didn't realize that I was moving her from a very poor environment to a very rich one, as well. We didn't even have a car, we didn't have a TV, we didn't have a computer, we were just poor.

Here, Nelly Coyote pauses and smiles warmly at me, and in her soft, gentle voice says,

But we weren't poor, you see, because I had had a lot of experiences. And I had friends I was real careful to keep in touch with, so we had people to visit. Then people came to see me, and we had books, and she was a great reader. That's why she got financial aid to go to RRPS—because she could do so well on the tests and everything. But for material things, we didn't have much. And they had a whole lot there! At RRPS, she made two special friends that she's still friends with. One of them's father puts $20,000 in her checking account every month—that's how rich they are! And that's nothing! They buy her a car when she needs one, and they go anywhere and do anything they want. They're really rich! . . . But, anyway, so that's one of her friends, and the other friend is not that rich, but her mother's a doctor so that's a lot richer than Liza was or even could have been. Her daddy was Black, and he grew up without any money at all. Everything they did was barter when he was growing up, and he, as far as he was concerned, he made it because he got land which Liza inherited, and in that community, he was looked up to as someone who had made it. . . .

But it's made her really smart because the people who belong in that environment, like RRPS, they don't know poor people. They don't know that we're real even. They have a lot of stereotypes and things, but they don't really know, whereas Liza knows both. So, she did okay. She did okay. She knows. I remember one time she was in a little group; they were making a video at RRPS, and I had to take her to a certain friend's house; they were going to work on [the project]. We drove up to this place—when I finally found it! It was so big; it was enormous! It was so big that Liza could not get out of the car. And I said, "I know what you mean." It was so big, and they had one child! She had a whole wing of her own and everything. . . . That was a mind-blowing thing, and it made Liza—she had to do a lot of adjusting, of course. And it made her look—we've smoothed it out now— but for a while . . . she looked at me and her father and thought, well, why hadn't we done better? Why weren't we successful like the parents of the people she's going to school with? And to us, her daddy and I, we had been successful. I felt successful, and I still feel very lucky. I'd never dreamed I was going to own my own home and love it so much. So, to us, we are successful, but not compared to people like her friend.

And those people, they always go to private universities, and Liza did too! She just went right along. . . . The different colleges competed to get her because, for their statistics, I guess. In RRPS, they're such liberal, open-minded people—they're educated to be that way—people were prejudiced against her, but it was not blatant. But I do remember this one time they were having a group discussion, and they were discussing trying to get people from [a predominantly poor and minority neighborhood in the city] into RRPS, whatever, just something like that, and one guy said, "They can't come here, some of those people live on $10,000 a year." And Liza said, "Well, they can join our group because we're all the weirdos." And then she came home and asked me how much we had a year, and it wasn't even $10,000! It's that thing she was aware of.

You know what Liza told me? She was with this family, [her friend from school's] family, and they have a house in Colorado, and they're going to go there for a week or two, and [go hiking in the] Rocky Mountains. So, they go to the grocery store and spend hundreds of dollars on food, and when it's time to pack up and leave, she said, "Mother, they threw it all away!" I said, "So why didn't you get it?" I couldn't believe she let them throw it all away. Threw away canned goods, everything. Hundreds of dollars, because they ate out, mostly. They didn't cook in that much. I was so upset I said, "Why didn't you get it?" She said, "Well, I didn't want to embarrass myself." I said, "Next time, you embarrass yourself and bring us some food home." Because when she was going to RRPS, it was rough. I had a part-time job, and I had a Social Security check from her daddy's Social Security. We ate from food banks, every food bank in [the city].

But, like, those people at RRPS, they are all thin, really thin. Why? Because one thing is, they can afford better food, and they have other rewards besides food. Food's not the thing. They also can travel, and they can—I have just now got to the point where I have any money I can spend as I like, that doesn't have to go to necessities. But they had that all along, so you don't focus on food so much. [Food] is just one of many things. It's just something they take for granted in a way that poor people—like these children that live [down the road] and that came over here to use the phone—their daddy's coming home [and they told me], "He's going to have a check, we're going to go get a whole case of [soda] pop." And I think, poor kids. To them, that's exciting, and no telling what else they're going to eat. But rich people, they have food. But I know how rich people are. I didn't never used to, but when my daughter went to RRPS, I realized, "Oh, there are really rich people around and they eat different." They do, they eat more expensively. They eat salad, and they eat fresh stuff, and they eat high-quality things . . . whereas poor people just eat. First of all, [poor people] concentrate on eating a lot, and then it's just cheap food, bread and potatoes. . . .

I have a friend who's Jewish, from Austin, and she came to see me one time, and we went to church. Everyone there was fat, and I was fat, and [my husband] was fat—everyone was fat, except my friend, she was not fat, and my little girl, Liza, she's a little girl then, she looked at [my friend] and she said, "[Friend's name] has bones." [Laughter] Then I realized at that moment, "Hey, she's right, [my friend] has bones, and none of the rest of us do!" I hadn't really thought about it before that, but I thought about it that day. If you look around, we are . . . I don't find it particularly attractive. I wish people were in shape. We used to be. There's "city white women" and "poor white women," like, the white women around here look the same as we do. But there isn't that difference with Indians because they are still fat, because they're still Indians. I have been around Indians in Los Angeles, and they had similar bodies like we do around here, like you do at home. You still are in your same culture, you're still with your same people, still eat the same way, you're still not rich, you're still—I don't know—you're still who you are.

After graduating college, Liza moved back to their small town and began taking in foster children as a way to keep busy. She eventually adopted River, whom Nelly Coyote tells me is "very obese" and "addicted to food." River, who is at school down the road when Nelly and I meet for our interview, is Choctaw and Mexican-American and in first grade. She weighed sixty pounds at the age of two when she moved into their home as a foster child. River's biological mother (Choctaw) struggles with drug use and "used to put her into a room with a bunch of food and lock her in all day." Because of this, Nelly Coyote says River is:

Obsessed with food—her mother was addicted to meth, and she hasn't been a happy child. She's been a depressed, violent child. She still has temper tantrums you wouldn't believe. She's had this being-overweight-thing, but she's real smart. I guess being overfed like that, it fed her brain. She's a smart girl. Emotionally she's all over the place, but she can read better than anyone else in her class already. She'll have to go to another school if she's going to have to be challenged at all.

Nelly Coyote has her eyes (and intentions) forward for River, hopeful and already considering ways to improve River's opportunities.

I selected Nelly Coyote's story of historical trauma for several reasons: First, she identifies boarding school attendance as particular experiences in her family's history that are associated with pain, loss, poor health, death, and lack of opportunity. There are myriad (individually experienced) personal reminders that she relates to historical trauma through her personal narrative. These include her perception of herself and her family members not fitting in with social expectations; personal and familial difficulties in life; personal and familial traumatic experiences; and microaggressions, particularly indignities and hostile, negative slights and insults related to her Indianness—especially her name—and socioeconomic status. Second, Nelly Coyote talks about multiple generations in her narrative, from her parents to her granddaughter, really allowing for a fluidity in understanding how historical trauma is called upon to connect and make sense of the present and across time as well. Indeed, the boarding school experiences of her parent's generation truly serve as background and contextual information for the many experiences of her life, her daughter's life, and the future imaginings of her granddaughter's life. Finally, her experiences of contemporary structural violence, specifically poverty (and especially rural poverty), serve as salient reminders of past injustice, particularly inequalities with life chances.

Nelly Coyote's narrative is especially powerful because she describes the many ways in which she moves in between the historical and structural constraints of her life. Her narrative is at once one of loss and one of resilience. She describes how the values of education were instilled in her parents' generation through the boarding schools—instilled and enforced in the most heinous ways—and she took this value of education and used it as a counterweight to the dominant oppressive historical trauma narrative of boarding schools, evident in how she sent Liza to RRPS and is thinking about River's future education as well. To ensure that Liza had better opportunities, Nelly Coyote relocated to the city, lived impoverished at the margins of society, and pushed against the constraints of her life. In this way, she brings to life messages of resilience and passes them on to her daughter, who in fact did go on to college, is multilingual, constructs homes, has adopted a daughter, and is capable of making opportunities (both locally and non-locally) for herself. Important, too, is that Nelly Coyote was sure to maintain relationships throughout her life—a back-and-forth reciprocity that is a strong value in Indian communities—calling on others and collective resources as a way to move beyond what was/is available to her, again pushing against the structural constraints as a way to improve her and her daughter's lives. This shows yet another act of resilience in the midst of injustice and is highlighted as occurring *in spite of* the many challenges of her life. The following touching quote of Nelly Coyote's illustrates the hope and resiliency in the life she has created and will pass forward:

> River, the other day in the morning, she told me, "I haven't figured out what my purpose in the family is." I couldn't—I didn't know how to tell her either. I was thinking, how am I going to help her with this? Then that evening she said, "Well, I've got it all figured out." I said, "What have you got figured out now?" She said, "Well, Mama's purpose is to be strong and to teach us to be a strong family. Your purpose, Grandma, is to have love and be kind to everyone, and I've figured out my purpose!" I said, "What's your purpose?" She said, "My purpose is to be happy, and to keep being happy, and to be myself."

To me, Nelly Coyote smiled and asked, "Isn't that great?"

Understanding Historical Trauma in Embodied Heritage

Unpacking the embodied heritage framework requires that we evaluate the social realities of women's lives. Indeed, attending to these social and individual dimensions of their lives is what makes this a study of heritage and health, as opposed to a microcosmic study of the obesity "epidemic" among Indigenous peoples. In doing so, I have highlighted commonly reported themes of historical trauma in women's narratives to reveal how historical trauma is understood to feed and interact with contemporary experiences of structural violence and is called upon as a way of understanding health and wellbeing.

To understand the tangled and complex ways Choctaws link contemporary forms of violence and inequities with past traumatic events, I utilize Mohatt and colleagues' (2014) heuristic of historical trauma as public narrative. Through examination of these narrative themes, the macro-level historical, political-economic, and social inequalities that facilitate these micro-level experiences of oppression and injustice become clearer. For example, loss of cultural knowledge and the breakdown of families resulting from forced attendance at Indian boarding schools played a powerful role in cultivating the conditions in which women expressed a sense of social and cultural detachment. At the same time, women described everyday struggles with economic insecurity, family discord, and living in depleted environments. They communicated their anxieties associated with loss of culture, lack of respect for elders, and the prevalence of alcoholism and drug addiction, diabetes, and other indicators of poor health. Additionally, many of the women associated contemporary foodways—especially the commodities food program and other indicators of food insecurity—with relocation, removal (the Trail of Tears), and historical losses of land, farming and gardening, and Indigenous knowledges. However, narratives of historical trauma also serve as stories of resistance and resiliency in which women identify the injustices of the past and the ways in which they give shape and meaning to their present experiences; they use these stories and understandings as touchstones for ongoing resistance: "And yet, we are still here." Understanding these multiple intersections is critical because the confluence of historical trauma, structural violence, and poverty—and the ways in which people make sense of these experiences—contribute to the significant burdens of obesity and food insecurity within this population.

Nelly Coyote used the phrase "a secret way of being" to call upon the exhausted existence of indigeneity. Sammy referred to "going Indian" and "shutting down" as a response to what Belcourt describes as the "conditions under which life is haphazardly improvised," where you constantly must just "make do," effecting a physical fragility and an intellectual fatigue that "circumscribes the body's potentialities" (Belcourt 2018:3). What is notable is that many of the women spoke about historical trauma and loss not as abstract, removed events, necessarily located in the past. Rather, they spoke about historical trauma and loss as if they were speaking about these traumatic events and losses happening *now*, affecting loved ones *today*, evoking grief and pain felt in the present. For example, Sherry from chapter 2 told me explicitly, "I don't like to read or talk about the history of Indians, like the Trail of Tears. I don't like hearing a thing about that because I get really sick. . . . I realize it's in the past, and that our people came through it, but . . ." Sherry stopped there and began to cry. She hunched over and held herself tightly, "If it was just left alone, but they don't leave it alone! It comes up all the time." Weeping, she forced out those last words, attempting to rationalize her emotions, her *felt* knowledge, as simply a product of overexposure to conversations about historical events. Nelly also described her mother's reaction to discussions about the Trail of Tears: Her mother too would cry and appear to be in physical pain, so much so that, as a child, Nelly believed that her mother had walked the Trail of Tears *herself*, because her pain and loss was so present, immediate, and intense.

The visceral way in which these women experience and articulate historical trauma—where the past is not distanced but deeply felt in the present—shows how their embodied knowledge disrupts settler-colonial time, rejecting the notion that trauma is confined to the past and instead asserting its ongoing presence in contemporary life. This is also recognizable in the ways that the women's narratives weave together the past, present, and future with modes of settler violence, becoming, in Mark Rifkin's (2017:33) words, "intimate parts of indigenous temporalities," but done so as "part of Native frames of reference, meaning that they are encountered through a perceptual tradition and a set of material inheritances that include ongoing Indigenous legacies of landedness, mobility, governance, ritual periodicities, social networks, and intergenerational stories." Rifkin argues that these myriad aspects of *being* and *becoming* together give historical density to the engagement with settler policies and everyday presence and, furthermore, orient Native perception and action. In these ways, historical trauma as public narrative can be understood both as a useful heuristic of how historical trauma "works" (i.e., present experiences of disenfranchisement recall historical experiences, which in turn influence how [and to what degree] people link the present with the past) *but also as* an example of Indigenous temporalities that challenges a settler-imposed linear temporality. As one woman told me, "The past is always with us; how can it not be? Just look at those rocks," referring to striations common in the area. "You see layers and layers of the past right here, all together. You can see the past, touch it, *feel* it. The past is always here."

Indeed, Nelly Coyote, Sammy, Sherry, and the other women feel the historical trauma and loss brought forth in the moment of their telling. Dian Million's work on felt knowledge theory underscores the importance of including lived experience, rich with emotional knowledges, and makes the case for experiences of individual and communal pain as a point of analysis that recognizes emotion as an embodied knowledge. Felt knowledge (Million 2009) often accompanies oral tradition, carried across and within temporalities alongside stories, knowledges, and traditions. For these women, experiences of misery—particularly as they relate to health—are not just personal afflictions; they are deeply embedded in what it means to be Indian within their communities. This suffering reflects relational dimensions of identity shaped by a collective imagination of indigeneity grounded in the lived realities of social, political, and economic marginalization. These notions of "being Indian" are not abstract; they manifest as embodied effects of structural violence that impact individuals and reverberate across entire communities. Such experiences of pain and affect are not merely symptoms to be therapeutically managed but are forms of felt knowledge—a kind of felt theory that registers the historical and ongoing conditions of colonial dispossession (Million 2009). Rather than pathologizing Indigenous experiences through psychological frameworks alone, this work situates historical trauma within a broader matrix of structural harm, where embodiment itself becomes a site of both memory and resistance.

By emphasizing how contemporary experiences of food insecurity, economic hardship, and health disparities are linked to the forced attendance at boarding schools, land loss, and settler policies, historical trauma as narrative underscores how colonial systems produce the very conditions of suffering. Moreover, instead of reinforcing neoliberal governance strategies that promote resilience as an individual responsibility (as Million rightfully warns against), these women's narratives expose the root causes of suffering, linking present-day struggles to a long history of structural dispossession. This framework also moves beyond symbolic recognition to create space for material reparations and decolonization. The women's reflections on food insecurity, for instance, do not just highlight the impact of trauma on health but point directly to settler policies—such as the commodities food program and forced agricultural shifts—that continue to shape Indigenous health and well-being. By connecting their experiences of poverty and violence to the history of land removal and assimilation policies, these narratives make an explicit demand for structural change rather than merely seeking therapeutic relief.

Finally, obesity affects these women's lives, placed not necessarily at the center of their stories but as intersecting conditions, symbiotic with other life experiences of being Indian. Their stories also reflect heterotemporality: multiple temporal formations with as many multiple ways of experiencing time. Meaning-making as a temporal orientation for these women reveals divergent processes of becoming and unbecoming. Their stories of the past and the present create situations for recollections in the future, helping to (re)shape collective memory and public narrative. As Rifkin notes, "Being temporally oriented suggests that one's experiences, sensations, and possibilities for action are shaped by the existing inclinations, itineraries, and networks in which one is immersed, turning toward some things and away from others. . . . It involves reiterated and nonconscious tendencies, suggesting ways of inhabiting time that shape how the past moves toward the present and future."

This points to resistance, too, as their narratives situate their individual experiences within the larger constructs of historical trauma and contemporary everyday violences. Their stories remind us to look beyond notions of victimhood and failure to understanding the more complex narratives of Indian people and communities that neither ignore the larger settler-colonial context nor focus singly on the continued existence of Indians in the face of settler-colonialism. For these women, historical trauma is put to work as a political act against erasure and individual responsibility. It calls attention to the invisible social machinery of structural violence and oppression, shifting inquiries surrounding obese bodies away from medical, public health, or lifestyle (behavior) discourses to political-economic and socio-cultural ones. Historical trauma as a public narrative calls for recognition that contemporary experiences of obesity and related health conditions are not isolated or ahistorical; they are embedded within a longer continuum shaped by the ongoing structures of settler colonialism.

An embodied heritage framework that includes historical trauma as public narrative allows for an understanding of the ways historical trauma narratives work to reconcile the past in the present and trauma with resiliency, as well as the ways in which women at once remember the past while engaged in the present. Historical trauma as public narrative allows for active agency and makes space for a deeper analysis, allowing for a greater understanding of historical trauma narratives as active, living sites of meaning-making, representation, and purposeful engagement for individuals and communities. These women are Indigenous storytellers, not merely recounting their pain, but sharing their lived experiences to resist erasure, to reclaim their histories, to affirm Indigenous survival, and to offer a means of countering settler narratives that can only ever recognize Indigenous trauma (but never demand redress). Historical trauma as public narrative allows for ongoing acts of defiance, exposing the ongoing machinery of settler colonialism, clearing space for better understandings of how larger historical and structural factors figure into social processes, individual health, *and* how people make sense of these connections. In the next chapter, I explore women's experiences of symbolic and everyday violence, as well as heritage-making within our understanding of historical trauma narratives, as a way to more fully examine processes of meaning-making that are at the heart of the embodied heritage framework.

CHAPTER 4

Heritage, Embodied

A Space for Meaning-Making

On a sunny and oppressively humid May morning, hundreds of Choctaws park their cars at Wheelock Academy in Garvin, Oklahoma, and board Choctaw Casino Resort shuttle buses to Millerton City Park, not quite three miles away. Right after ten o'clock, *Minko* (*Chahta* for "Chief") Gary Batton addresses the crowd with quick pleasantries and a reminder to reflect not only on our ancestors but on the women and men serving our country today as well. He hands the microphone over to Reverend Curtis, who leads the crowd in a prayer, after which organizers begin playing the Lord's Prayer in *Chahta anumpa* over mobile loudspeakers. Three Choctaw princesses, wearing Choctaw dresses and tall beaded crowns, move in *Chahta* sign language along to the Lord's Prayer, their hands and bodies flowing with the hymn, translating *Chahta* with their movements.[1] The crowd's attention is then directed toward the Choctaw Nation Color Guard in their red berets and shouldered rifles, who carry both the U.S. and Choctaw Nation of Oklahoma flags as they take the first steps to signal the beginning of the Trail of Tears Commemorative Walk.[2]

The trail traced that day is not part of the original Trail of Tears, but it is on a dirt road, rocky and sometimes difficult to traverse. Those walking (or being pushed in wheelchairs) are carrying bananas, Gatorade, apple juice, and water bottles and wearing baseball caps and sunglasses. Water stations are set up along the way, and medics and transportation are available to anyone in need. The dust from the road puffs around footsteps, sticking to sweaty skin and sneaking into eyes, nostrils, and skin crevices. The walk begins solemnly and quietly, the only sound the clinking of pebbles and the crunching of dirt under shoes. Murmurs of conversation slowly rise, and as folks move deeper into the walk—legs, arms, and steps swaying in rhythms—people start talking, sharing, and connecting. Silence becomes chatter; chatter becomes conversations; conversations becomes laughter. One woman from Texas, pushing her eighty-year-old mother in a wheelchair, describes that while walking past small creeks, she thinks about her ancestors walking through rivers and the drownings along the Trail of Tears she has heard about. For her, physically walking in this event evokes heartbreaking mental imagery of Choctaws, walking, having lost everything. But she simultaneously holds that pain with the knowledge that her ancestors kept going, putting one foot in front of the other until they reached their new home. A man walking nearby overhears the conversation and chimes in, saying simply, "Determination." He participates in the commemorative walk every year because this act of remembering makes him feel "free" and "determined." He says he never misses the annual walk because he needs to do what his ancestors did; he needs to feel what his ancestors felt so he can feel "free" and be willing to do more, not just for others, but for himself too. This event—the walking, the dirt road, the people, the remembering, the conversations—is a living, moving site of profound complexity: It is both the meaning-making around the pain and devastation of the historical event, actively remembered—in multiple ways—*and* a way in which resistance and resilience are crafted, seemingly across a continuum. At one end, resistance is attested simply through being alive today as survivors of that traumatic event. At the other end, resistance is resiliency, illustrated through feelings of *determination* and *freedom*, reflecting current conditions of inequality in which people tap into their histories as a way to garner strength to carry on. A common sentiment is, "If our ancestors survived *that*, we can survive *this*."[3]

When the walkers reach Wheelock Academy, about an hour later, the Nation has set up tents with tables and chairs. Burgers and hot dogs are on the grills, and vendors are selling t-shirts, trinkets, and beadwork. A band has just begun playing covers of popular country music, and walkers are slowly arriving. As soon as everyone is there, having either completed the walk or been picked up by one of the vehicles, Minko Batton stands on the makeshift stage to address the crowd. First, however, he asks all the diabetics to raise their hands so that the crew can be sure to feed them first. Nearly half of the crowd raises a hand.

The first Trail of Tears Commemerative Walk I attended, I had trouble processing what I felt were contradictions. For example, the location, the grounds where we were commemorating the Trail, was Wheelock Academy, a missionary boarding school with a history of abusing children for speaking *Chahta*.[4] This was coupled with a BBQ-party vibe to the lunch afterward. It all felt counter to a commemoration of the Trail of Tears, arguably the most devastating historical event for our people. I struggled with this feeling of celebration, which seemed sort of inappropriate, until I realized that this was the point. The range of activities in this commemoration include remembering (and embodying that remembering), commemorating, communicating, and passing on knowledge and memories, but also asserting and expressing identity, relationality, and social and cultural values and meanings (Smith 2006). New memories are also being created. This is significant for Choctaw youth who become enveloped in new collective memories passed on from elders, but also everyone gains new memories through the process of being at the walk while also negotiating new meanings about what it means to "be" at the walk. As an experience and as a social and cultural performance, then, the Trail of Tears Commemorative Walk creates (and continually recreates) social networks and relations that come together and create a sense of belonging and identity around, specifically, resiliency. It is a celebration of survival that is actively (re)created and negotiated as Choctaws reinterpret, remember, and reassess meanings of the past in terms of the social, cultural, and political needs of the present. Further, it is as much about the future—where we are going—as it is about the past—where we have come from.

Today, the commemorative walk is held in *Tvshka Homma* (Tuskahoma), the former capitol of the Choctaw Nation and the location of the Chahta Village, a permanent structure replicating traditional *chukka* (homes). The walk is two and a half miles around the capitol grounds and ends in the Chahta Village, where demonstrations of traditional activities and food tastings are available. At the 2017 event, the organizers hung banners of quotes from Chief George Harkins' *Letter to the American*

People, including, for example, "We as Choctaws rather chose [sic] to suffer and be free, than live under the degrading influence of laws, which our
voice could not be heard in their formation," and "I could cheerfully hope,
that those of another age and generation may not feel the effects of those
oppressive measures that have been so illiberally dealt out to us; and that
peace and happiness may be their reward."[5] I have come to recognize that
the Trail of Tears Commemorative Walk is simultaneously about creating
and maintaining historical and social memory of Choctaw suffering *and*
a process of dissent and contestation. Specifically, it contests both that
Choctaws are merely victims and that suffering is in the past (as evident,
for example, by the number of diabetics in the crowd). The Trail of Tears
Commemorative Walk is a cultural process and performance, a heritage
process, that is about the negotiation of these conflicts. Smith (2006:82)
argues, "Heritage *is* dissonant—it is a constitutive social process that on
the one hand is about regulating and legitimizing, and on the other hand
is about working out, contesting and challenging a range of cultural and
social identities, sense of place, collective memories, values and meanings that prevail in the present and can be passed to the future."

In this chapter, I present the major themes around the social processes of heritage and identity described in women's life stories, complemented with a deeper understanding of meaning-making, which is
the heart of the embodied heritage framework and demonstrates how
women's experiences figure into the promulgation of obesity and identity
among Choctaws. The chapter begins with an overview of what Laurajane Smith (2006) has called the "authorized heritage discourse," which
privileges expert values over those of community and local interests and
which works to constrain understandings of heritage as primarily material. Then, I present the conceptualization of heritage used in this framework and describe how it interacts with identity. Next, I unpack the most
prevalent experiences that women described in their food-centered life
history narratives related to Indianness (markers of identity) and notions
of heritage. Finally, based on analysis of their stories, I demonstrate how
meaning-making illuminates the ways in which larger structural factors
figure into social processes and individual health and how people make
sense of these connections in the construction of cultural identity. This
chapter demonstrates how an embodied heritage framework under-
stands health as shaped by one's social, economic, historical, cultural,

and political context, as well as by the interpretive structures that give meaning to lived, bodily experience.

Heritage

In her book *The Uses of Heritage*, archeologist Laurajane Smith (2006) problematizes what she calls the *authorized heritage discourse*—a historically, institutionally, and politically situated discourse that identifies sites, places, buildings, and artifacts that heritage "experts" claim as monumental, grand, valuable, aesthetic, old, and importantly, "heritage for all." The authorized heritage discourse is the dominant view of heritage. It is how heritage has been defined and talked about among scholars and experts for years, arguing ultimately for preservation (Harvey 2008; Smith 2006). It focuses attention on aesthetically pleasing material culture, such as objects, sites, places, or landscapes, that current generations must care for, protect, and revere so that they may be passed on to future generations (Harrison 2009; Smith 2003, 2006). The authorized heritage discourse holds that the value of material culture is *innate* rather than *associative*. In this discourse, *heritage* is understood as fragile, finite, and non-renewable, rationalizing who or which "experts" are best suited to protect, understand, and communicate the value of heritage to others (Graham and Howard 2008; Harrison 2009; Smith 2006). These experts include archaeologists, anthropologists, architects, historians, museum curators, and heritage managers, whose power and knowledge claims strengthen and legitimize the hegemonic heritage discourse to reflect "the grand narratives of nation and aesthetics . . . establish[ing] who has the power or 'responsibilities' to define and 'speak for' the past [while also creating and recreating] a range of social relations, values and meanings about both the past and present" (Smith 2006:42). In Indigenous communities, these "experts" rarely include the community members themselves. Thus, the authorized heritage discourse promotes a static and preserved notion of heritage, and consequently, heritage *is* the monument (or other material thing or place) rather than the cultural values or meanings (Smith 2003, 2006).

Searching for a way to include alternate discourses in the field of heritage, Smith (2006:44) argues that "heritage is not a 'thing,' it is not a 'site,' building or other material object. . . . Heritage is what goes on at these sites. . . . [Heritage] is a cultural process that engages with acts of remembering that work to create ways to understand and engage with the present." In her work with the Waanyi women in Australia on heritage sites in the Boodjamulla National Park (2003), she recognized that heritage was *being experienced* at these sites; in fact, this was a requirement for a site to be considered "heritage" among the Waanyi women. In other words, *heritage is the experience.* Smith argues that heritage is active, action, alive, and includes remembering, commemorating, passing on memories and knowledge, meaning-making, expressing and asserting identity, and social and cultural values and meanings. Heritage produces emotions, experiences, and memories that can foster a sense of belonging and identity and social relations that create and recreate a sense of belonging and identity—identities that are constantly negotiated and recreated through the processes of remembering and making meaning of the past as it serves the present. Put simply, heritage is the "process of remembering that underpins identity and the ways in which individuals and groups make sense of their experiences in the present" (Smith 2006:276). Importantly, heritage is an active process (Dicks 2000; Graham and Howard 2008; Lowenthal 1998; Smith 2006). It is an active process that is found in the banal of everyday life, including "just being together" and eating food together. This is a critical point, as the goal of this research is to understand not only *what* Choctaws identify as heritage, but *why*, *how*, and *when* this heritage-making occurs, and furthermore how it dialectally interacts with human biologies and health.

This revised conceptualization of heritage refocuses attention from the material fabric of heritage to those who use it. Meaning-making is an important part of heritage, as it touches on the many aspects of heritage: what it is, what it does, and what it means to individuals and groups. In asking how people make meaning, we are also asking "why? What is it that is being sought from heritage?" Smith (2006:125), acknowledging that individuals are not mere passive receivers of heritage but rather active constructors of heritage, argues that we must ask, "What is the cultural, political and social work that heritage does?" If *heritage* is the contemporary usage of the past, or an active processing of the past, then different meanings of the past give space for contestation and lack of consensus over heritage. Tunbridge and Ashworth (1996:27) call this "dissonant heritage," arguing that ". . . all heritage is someone's heritage and therefore logically not someone else's: the original meaning of an inheritance (from which 'heritage' derives) implies the existence of disinheritance and by extension any creation of heritage from the past disinherits someone completely or partially, actively or potentially . . ." This notion of *dissonant heritage* is useful in this research, as it relates to the process of coping with ambivalent and largely unwanted pasts, such as the Trail of Tears or other events of historical trauma.

The purpose of meaning-making, particularly among those with dissonant heritage, is to identify the main elements of an event (e.g., loss of language and knowledge of other traditional cultural expressions from boarding schools) and integrate those experiences into a coherent personal narrative (Joseph and Linley 2005; Park and Ali 2006). That is indeed what happens in Indian communities with historical trauma, especially when historical trauma is called upon as public narrative. Narrative, in its many forms then, can be seen as central to heritage (Bendix 2002; Chronis 2011; Watson and Waterton 2010) and has been widely used in heritage research (Adabala et al. 2010; Edelheim 2015; Ramshaw 2014), indicating that heritage narratives are not only an essential ingredient in the construction of personal, collective, and place identities, but are also important in the process of contemplating, experiencing, and remembering heritage experiences. Furthermore, meaning-making from narratives, particularly trauma narratives, is argued to be a mechanism of healing, because the new knowledge or perspective garnered from this process transforms old beliefs into new ones that can now hold the experience without being too discrepant (Calhoun and Tedeschi 2014; Janoff-Bulman 2006). Narrative research with survivors of trauma illustrates that they continuously work to integrate past experiences into a coherent narrative as a way to better understand their present and future selves; thus, researchers argue that meaning-making is the mechanism for creating coherence (Bochner and Riggs, 2014; Josselson 2011). Understanding meaning-making that is part of heritage (or dissonant heritage), then, will aid in understanding the related elements of resilience. In the case of dissonant heritage, working with community reflections of historical trauma often results in community engagement practices, and it is the engagement with community around meaning-making of dissonant heritage that *is* the medicine that helps the community toward healing practices.

Finally, heritage can be understood as an important political and cultural tool in defining and legitimizing Choctaw ways of belonging, being in relation, and socio-cultural and political recognition. Likewise, heritage can be understood as an important resource in challenging *received* versions of these ways of belonging, being in relation, and different forms of recognition (Smith 2006).

Anthropology has long recognized *identity* as fluid, multiple, and socially constructed. Barth (1969) considers identity as the product of a complex process of constant (re)shaping, including ascription by others and self-categorization. This is compatible with notions of identity as contextual, such that an individual can identify with a group in certain situations and not in others (Barth 1969; Bucholtz and Hall 2004, 2005; Cohen 1986; Nagel 1999). Bucholtz and Hall (2004) argue that identity is realized in people's actions rather than a fixed list of traits, and it is intimately connected to the continuous responses of others, as well as appraisals of ourselves made by us and others (Frideres 2008; Ochs and Capps 1996). Identity is also constructed by macro-processes, outside agents, and organizations that (re)shape categories and definitions (Cornell 1988; Jaimes 1992; McBeth 1989; Nagel 1999). In critical Indigenous studies, the concept of *identity* is heavily critiqued for offering a limiting and individualist framework that fails to capture the deeply relational ways in which Indigenous peoples understand themselves; it is perceived as an imposed construct rooted in settler colonial logics of classification and personal self-definition rather than Indigenous ways of being that are fundamentally relational, shaped by kinship, land, and community (TallBear 2019; Simpson 2014, 2017). I use the term *identity* with caution, recognizing the potential danger it can inflict by reducing Indigenous belonging to questions of self-identification or legal recognition, and follow Indigenous scholars who push for a shift from identity to relationality as an ongoing practice of lived relationships, responsibilities, and participation in Indigenous lifeways, always rooted in community and accountability to human and non-human kin, land, and traditions (Byrd 2011; Coulthard 2014; Simpson 2014, 2017; TallBear 2019; Todd 2016; Tuck and Yang 2012; Watts 2013). This relational practice (i.e., identity) is an active process, and the links between identity and heritage can be expressed in multiple ways: actively or passively within the authorized heritage discourse, in active opposition to the authorized heritage discourse, or in less self-conscious ways constructed outside of (or without reference to) the authorized heritage discourse (Smith 2006).

Heritage means different things to different people. In the next section, I present findings from the food-centered life history interviews that illustrate a slipperiness and dissonance of what is understood to be heritage (e.g., Graham et al. 2000; Loulanski 2006; Tunbridge and Ashworth 1996). For many Choctaws, heritage is used to describe traditions and knowledge such as *Ishtaboli* (stickball),[6] basket weaving, weapon-making, cultural dances, certain foods, stories, songs, and "just being together." Choctaws also refer to another type of heritage: the heritage of violence that has led to current conditions of poor health, poverty, and loss of land and food sovereignty (Farmer 1999; Quesada et al. 2011). Choctaw notions of heritage are two sides of the same coin: Honoring traditional cultural expressions inherently invokes the painful histories of forced removal, assimilation, cultural suppression, and dispossession. These intertwined aspects of heritage are inseparable and self-referential: The presence of one inevitably calls forth the other.

Women's Narratives of Heritage

The women in this study often first referred to traditional cultural expressions such as speaking *Chahta anumpa*, playing *Ishtaboli* (stickball), or wearing Choctaw clothing as the easiest way to relay their Choctaw heritage. These expressions distinguish Choctaws from non-Choctaws, including from other tribal citizens, and serve as material culture symbolic not only of their identities, but of certain values as well. Furthermore, they are chosen and adorned specifically to do so. For example, one woman described intentionally wearing clothing and accessories with recognizable Choctaw symbols, such as beaded caps, lanyards, diamond patterned headbands, or t-shirts that indicate involvement in the Choctaw Nation. Living in southeastern Oklahoma, many of the women want others to be able to discern that they are Choctaw, as opposed to being mistaken for Mexican or white.

Heritage, as we understand, is not just the material—it's what happens around the material. For many people, heritage also means markers such as "looking Indian," but that does not hold up when we unpack heritage. For example, one woman said that "being Choctaw is brown skin, dark brown eyes, and dark hair. Of course, if you speak the language—I can't, but . . . I guess learning the traditional ways and everything. But I don't know all the traditional ways, and I don't know how to speak the language. I just know I'm full-blood . . ." (Annette, Durant).

For many, heritage is the (re)creation of values of resiliency, adaptability, and determination, as described at the Trail of Tears Commemorative Walk. Women described overcoming challenges and hardship as a value they (re)create by reflecting on the past through the lens of their current positionalities. Billie, another woman I spoke with, described how struggle is something all Choctaws have experienced, but it is the response to struggle that reveals what *being Choctaw* is really about.

> To be Choctaw, it really means that my family had to struggle. And the fact that there is still a family line means that we were able to win. And that shows me that we have perseverance, and we're stubborn, and we have determination and willpower. I am proud to be Choctaw. I'm very proud to be a member of the Choctaw Nation . . . because staying with my grandmother during the days and everything, she'll tell me stories about when she was a child. Because she had to go to the [Indian boarding school] when she was four or five years old, and that was during the Indian round up that they did in this area, because my grandmother was born and raised in this area. And to hear about that and to hear all of the struggles that she had to go through, and that her father had to go through, it really hit home. Because nowadays, I don't know if I would be able to do everything that my family in the past had been able to do and accomplish. But it gives me hope that I will be able to do that . . . yeah. The way that we were able to prosper and pull ourselves up from the dirt because when the—everyone got pushed over here and the Trail of Tears happened. I don't think anyone really expected [our ancestors] to stand up like they did and prosper and grow. Because it could have very well been a deceased, extinct race. But because we do have that willpower and the strength—being Choctaw . . . that's what I think of, willpower, determination, strength. If you think you can do it, put your mind to it and do it. That's what "Choctaw" is to me. (Billie, Durant)

Heritage is just as much about the future as it is about the past. Most of the women in this research described being proud of these values, especially because they feel hopeful about the future and the Choctaw Nation's strength and advancement, another testament to their resiliency as individuals and as a collective.

> I didn't grow up learning or knowing about Choctaw culture or ways or history, but I learned it later on. And I think probably later on, I was more appreciative of who I was and what our Choctaw people went through and, like, everything that our ancestors done. I think knowing those things now, I have a deeper appreciation for my Choctaw ancestors and knowing that people before me did a lot of these things and accomplished all of these things and knowing that I have a lineage to that, and that does make me proud of who I am, just being a part of a significant group of individuals that made a huge contribution to the existence of who we are now today. Hopefully, we can pay our homage to our ancestors and continue to promote Choctaw culture, Choctaw ways to my generation and our future generations. That's what we try to do now with our kids, our nieces, our younger people, our younger relatives, and we have a grandson. So now it's important, more than ever, because our language is on the verge of being lost. Now we're trying to prevent that. We do speak Choctaw to him. He's only seven months old but I'm like, "The sooner we can get in there!" (Jenny, Broken Bow)

The women are grateful that the Choctaw Nation has continued its relational responsibility,[7] as indicated by the many services made available to tribal citizens, including housing, financial aid and counseling, transportation, healthcare, and especially foods through the Food Distribution Program. Women commented that it was "beneficial" to be Indian today, and indeed, feeling "proud" of their indigeneity is a newer sentiment expressed among the women in this project. It's a sentiment that is reinforced by their access to "benefits" while living among non-Choctaws who do not have access to these same "benefits" (services). This distinction is made all the more visible by the roads, stores, casinos, travel plazas, community centers, wellness centers, and now cattle ranches constructed, owned, and operated by the tribe. Tribal citizens have access to many services which their (also poor, but non-Choctaw) neighbors do not have access to. As Tracy describes below, the sense of *coming from nothing* and *taking care of each other* is Choctaw heritage.

> It wasn't so cool to be Native American, where now it is. Everybody wants it. Not everybody, I shouldn't say that. But I have lots of friends that'll say, "I just need a drop of blood. I just need one." And I get a lot of calls about how to find their ancestry, their roll number, their Dawes number.... I just feel so good that I have what I do. Anyway, it's pretty cool. There's more benefits. Before it weren't a benefit thing, where they didn't do things for you. Now we have some money, and they try to take care of our people to keep our culture alive. But I think a long time ago, well, not a long time, in the '40s, '50s, '60s . . . and it wasn't. (Tracy, Poteau)

The women I spoke with were really trying to pinpoint the banality of Choctaw heritage, or the "just being together" in the day-to-day that makes up what it means to be Choctaw. They described heritage as the process and interactions of daily *living, knowing,* and *being* together in family, among friends, in familiar settings, sites, and places in which so-cial and cultural values and meanings get passed on—in which Choctaws learn *how to be* Choctaws. Veronica eloquently describes this:

> To me, [heritage] is that you grew up a Choctaw. That you knew—you can sing in Choctaw. You went to the Indian churches, you had fellowship. You were neighborly. It wasn't anything to just pick up and go visit someone and be welcome there. And then someone to come see you and share what you have. It isn't anything like it is today. It's just a part of you, it's some-thing that you have inside you. It's not something that you adorn yourself with, or a dress, a Choctaw dress . . . My culture, because I guess I've been in a dominant society for so long that, although I have it within me and I know the values and the traditions, it's a segment of a society that really hardly exists—the actions. There's tones and overtones of doing things, the cultural activities and such, and going out to the masses and showing them how to weave a basket and then you're gone, but that's not living the cultural life. To me it's the values of sharing, and the compassion, and the willingness to help, the giving. All of those things are, to me, part of our culture and not just because you get paid [to perform it]. (Veronica, Durant)

If heritage is the process of remembering that underpins identity (or Indigenous relationality) and the ways in which people make sense of their experiences in the present (Smith 2006), then for Billie, Tracy, Veronica, and the other women in this research, "just being here" is a process of heritage: recognizing that "just being here"—when the goal of settler colonialism is elimination—is a cultural process that engages with acts of remembering that work to create ways to understand and engage with the present. Thus, struggle, hardship, and discrimination in the present (and the past) are tools that facilitate this process. Remembering is an active process in which the past both collectively or individually is continually negotiated and reinterpreted through, not only the experiences of the present, but also the needs of the present (Smith 2006; Wertsch 2011). For instance, health disparities among Choctaws is a pressing concern that demands more scrutiny; women in this research often called on the past as a way to make sense of contemporary experiences of all types of health concerns.

Carmen, for example, is a thirty-year-old woman who works at one of the community centers helping connect tribal citizens with tribal services. She had been diagnosed as obese and prediabetic and strongly advised by a doctor to lose weight or else suffer the consequences of her supposedly risky, faulty, fat body. Motivated not by her doctor's harsh words but instead by her upcoming wedding and desire to fit into her mother's wedding dress, Carmen lost a lot of weight—at least four pants sizes, she tells me—and shares one of her favorite childhood memories.

> We had lots of cousins, and they were always around; it was all of us. I remember some of us had [baby] bottles and maybe we were too old to have bottles because I can still remember one [cousin] that was taller than us didn't have a bottle, but she was—I guess we were whining or crying or something, playing and she would say, "I think they need their bottle refilled." And so, my aunty would say, "Well, help them." . . . And we would go to the kitchen, a herd of us would go in there and she would climb up on the sink, and I remember her turning on the water and rinsing our bottles out. She knew to do that, but she would reach into the sugar jar and put a deal of sugar in the bottle and put water in it. She would shake it, and she would call out your name because we'd already started playing and she would hand it out and we'd just wait for her and then she'd climb

down. She might do two or three bottles, and then we'd all follow her back in because she was a little bit older than us. And then my aunty would say, "Oh, you did good. You got them water and they're not crying." She was the big cousin taking care of us, she thought. I could remember thinking how much I loved that and getting excited about when I had seen them taking my bottle. If it was just water that would have been great for me. But I know I seen her putting sugar in it. Somebody taught her to do that.

Here, Carmen pauses for a moment, making a connection between this beloved memory of family, sugar-water bottles, and how she lives now. She continues:

But if we'd kept all of our traditions, continued to hunt, continued those practices passed down through generations before ours, then we wouldn't have diabetes and obesity. There's no additives and preservatives [in what we hunt], and it doesn't go to the meat market, and it doesn't . . . all that. My husband, he's full-blood Choctaw and he loves to hunt. Deer season, if he kills a deer, he wants to eat that deer meat that night. It's a family thing on his side, because there are a lot of Choctaws. If they're fishing . . . if he catches it that afternoon, they want to have fish fry. They want to cook up that fresh fish. It's different, their meat! It's so healthy for us because it's never been in the meat market, it's never going to get *E. coli*, it's not going to get touched by salmonella in the factory. They're not doing cesspools and making sausage and all this. They usually get all the deer guts and stuff and let the wild animals have a meal on it. It's healthy for [the animals] . . . And sometimes they use the antlers, they hang them outside if they go hunting. . . . They take it and hope it'll bring some deer. They just try to use everything they can and all the meat. If they get a good size[d deer] they give some to other families and then they freeze some and then, and there's nothing. I mean you can't get healthier than eating a deer that's running by because it has nothing, you know? . . .

They think they are vegetarian because they only eat fresh deer. And my husband, he's very healthy, because that's how he grew up. When they eat meat—and they eat a lot of deer meat—they just get it out of their freezer. When [I was growing up] we ate hamburger meat and stuff like that, you know how it's been to the meat market? He probably don't have half those things in his body because he grew up all fresh fish and deer meat and has all the best memories of that. When he gets ready to hunt, when he gets ready to fish, it's a ceremony for him. So, it just means that it's everything. I had to learn that because I never did eat deer meat until I met him. And I didn't use as much fish as I do now. It was hard at first. I would act like I would eat it, but I would put it in the trash [laughter]. Because it was hard for me to get the taste. He said it's because [I've] been eating processed meat, hamburger meat and store-bought stuff, and you have to get a taste for it. I have the taste for it now because I know it's so much more healthier. I watched it get packaged. I watched it get froze. I watched everything handled in a timely manner, versus all the news saying everything's got *E. coli* or bacteria and salmonella and recalling everything. He says, "They're not going to recall our meat."

Carmen's words—the stories she shares with me, the (dis)connections she draws between her own upbringing as a Choctaw woman and her husband's—offer insight into how personal and collective histories of trauma shape everyday understandings of identity and care. At other points in our interview, she shares about her family's history of Indian boarding school and the trauma they endured from growing up without their parents. Her aunty—the one who had been watching her and all the other little cousins—would talk about how hard it was to attend the school, how she and her brother and sister (Carmen's mom) would stick together, never left each other's sides since being sent to boarding school in first, second, and third grades. She would never share details of what the school was like for them but would talk about the relief and joy they felt over summers when they were reunited with their mom.

As she speaks, I am continually reminded of Belcourt's (2018:2) claim that "colonial affects escape analytic capture," moved by how easy it is to hear stories like Carmen's sugar-water bottles and think that the reservation is "bad for life because its members are bad *at* life." But Carmen's husband had a different experience. His family did not go to boarding school and were not subjected to the same violent assimilation policies. They kept their language, their ways of living and being in relation to land and each other. This is clear in her distinction between her foods and her husband's foods. His family eat deer from the rural woods, where deer consume local, organic plants that grow as intended, in relation with the land, other plants, and other non-humans; the deer roam unobstructed and live relationally, as they always have. In this family's understanding, they are "vegetarian" because when they consume the deer, they are consuming the vegetation that sustained the deer. The deer is not separate from its surroundings and is alive only because of the plants and larger ecosystems that sustain it. This viewpoint for sure complicates understandings of diet claims (e.g., vegetarianism) that center humans at the top of the "food chain" and focus on the singular (i.e., a plant, a deer, a root) rather than the holism of foodways, but it also recognizes a radical relationality that comes from Choctaw original teachings and recognition of (and responsibility to) the interdependence of all entities—human, land, water, and non-humans.

This gets at that heritage of the everyday; it gets at the ways in which memory is an active process, where the past—both collective and individual—is continuously renegotiated and reinterpreted through the lens of present experiences (obesity, diabetes, poor health) and needs (healthier foods, Choctaw foods). What's more, it gets at the dual reality of heritage for Choctaws whereby Carmen's husband has access to and knowledge of Choctaw foodways because his family evaded boarding schools. Carmen's family, on the other hand, grew up on plastic-wrapped ground beef and sugar water, severed from the knowledge that once sustained them. Yet, both are Choctaw, and to recognize Choctaw heritage is to acknowledge both survival and loss; even when celebrating what has carried forward, it is always in reference to what was taken. This is the heritage of the everyday—a dual reality where the good is inseparable from the bad, and remembering is always an act of reckoning.

Dissonant Heritage

Even within what is widely considered Choctaw heritage, there is dissonance. The tribe has recently and energetically pushed forward Choctaw culture and heritage, making efforts to provide classes on language, beading, basket weaving, moccasin making, and more. Notably, most of the older participants commented that what the tribe is teaching today, specifically *Chahta anumpa*, stories, and some of the dancing, is not what they grew up with. They discussed *Chahta anumpa* as being the most dissonant. Many of the women who speak *Chahta*, especially the older women, described that, as students in the language classes offered by the tribe, they often taught the teachers how to pronounce words "the right way" or corrected their sentence structure. One woman described how not only is the language "not quite right," but that a certain type of heritage narrative is being created around Wheelock Academy that does not sit well with her.

> I don't know. I can't speak for all the older ones, but they were like, "No, we didn't do that. That's not how we were—boarding schools, there weren't boarding schools." Boarding schools were mean to them, bad memories, and you want to celebrate Wheelock? Everybody that goes to Wheelock will come back, [saying] great times. It might have been great times for some, but for some, they were really bad times. That's what they remember about a long time ago and so you might have a lot of older ones that have negative thoughts about a lot of things that are going on. Even the language! That's not how they spoke, it's different. They're bringing in a different language.... They say it's the Mississippi, the way the Mississippi Choctaws talk, and they're bringing it down here, but that's not how they talk down here. (Mandy, Durant)

The tribe has invested a large amount of money to restore Wheelock Academy, and it now offers a museum that showcases, for example, what schoolrooms looked like during operation. They also have held meetings and other types of cultural gatherings at Wheelock, which have been met with opposition from some. Mandy commented that many of the elders were appalled that gatherings were held at this location, arguing that it seemed like the tribe was trying to rewrite the narrative of Wheelock, "probably because they now own it." Several women commented also that "Heritage Mondays," held the first Monday of every month at the CNO capitol, are showcases of culture that are sometimes inappropriate. For example, employees, many of whom are not Choctaw, are encouraged to wear traditional Choctaw clothing. However, some women argued that these clothes are (culturally) reserved for special occasions such as weddings or celebrations. To wear them to work, especially if the wearer is not Choctaw, can be seen as offensive and disrespectful.

We have employees here that are non-Indian that are wearing Choctaw dresses on Heritage Monday and I think, "Oh gosh, that's not a fitting situation to wear Choctaw tribal dress." So those types of things are occurring, you know, that it's becoming very common, where Choctaw dresses were saved for the best, the best of things. Like, my daughter and my sons, when we baptized them, my little daughter wore a Choctaw dress, and my sons wore the traditional Choctaw shirts. Those were what we considered the best clothes they had. . . . That was our best dress, that is a meaningful dress, that's what I would think. . . . I don't like [that non-Choctaws] wear these clothes. I absolutely don't like it. Because they've inserted themselves into—and I'm sure they're all well-intentioned. (Rosalie, Durant)

Sandra, a middle-aged woman from Broken Bow, said, "when the culture started coming," referring to the tribe's (re)introduction of traditional cultural expressions and how many of these expressions were previously unknown and are unrecognizable. Sandra described herself as "full-blood Choctaw," and her grandparents were well-known throughout the region for their service to other Choctaws. Her grandfather often delivered church sermons in *Chahta anumpa*, and her grandmother was highly regarded for driving folks around, feeding others, and making herself available. Sandra described how she was completely unaware of *Ishtaboli* (its practice was stopped for quite some time) as Choctaw heritage, but also how much of what is considered traditional Choctaw expressions was unknown to her, unrecognizable, or she could not remember it. I find it striking how she referred to the culture "coming," indicating simultaneously the efforts of the tribe to bring forth these expressions, as well as prompting one to wonder what it was like before "the culture started coming." She explained:

To me, I grew up in [rural town] my whole life. Choctaws to me were my family. We were Indian. We'd see other families and all this, but I didn't really know what the "Choctaw culture" was. My family was Choctaw, my grandma and grandpa would go to churches and speak. He was a minister and just every Sunday we would go to churches, different churches. He would talk and that's where Indians went, to camp meetings, weekends. To me, that was "Choctaw" growing up. . . . When the culture started coming,

I remember them doing dances—that was when [a local woman] and all of them, they were younger, and they were bringing in all these dancers. I used to dance a long time ago when I was little. And stickball! I didn't know nothing about stickball until they started coming out with it, what five or six years ago, if even that long ago. I didn't know nothing about that. I didn't even know we played it. I just knew the Choctaws were civilized. I didn't know they had these dances—I knew they danced but they weren't wild dances or anything—and they wore clothes. I don't remember them wearing feathers or anything like that or their traditional dances like they do. I didn't know nothing about that.

The Choctaw Nation has made great efforts to revitalize traditional cultural expressions as part of its tribal identity, offering language and beading classes, investing in stickball fields and training camps, showcasing heritage at almost every event, and offering cultural outreach and presentations to professional conferences, schools, and Daughters of the American Revolution, for example. They have completely revamped their website and now include multiple pages of information dedicated to Choctaw history and culture, stating, "We pride ourselves on preserving and celebrating our many *unique* traditions. From our *distinctive* language to our *historical* games, like stickball, to our *native* dances and artwork, we not only want to pass these *traditions* on to our youth, we want to share them with all people" (CNO 2018, emphasis mine). Note the words "unique," "distinctive," "historical," and "native" included in this description of the Nation's history and culture, words that often do not match up with the women's notions and recollections of Choctaw cultural expressions.

To understand what these women describe as a sort of "reinvention" of Choctaw heritage, it is necessary to understand Oklahoma heritage. Choctaws are identified as one of the Five "Civilized" Tribes in Oklahoma for adopting settler ways—that is, for being agriculturalists, for establishing schools, having written laws and a government, and adopting Christianity. This, coupled with more than a century of assimilation, cultural suppression, and loss of land and food sovereignty, represents the quality of being adaptable—something Choctaws have prided themselves on. Indeed, Choctaw adaptability is recognized as resiliency, and both are fundamental values of Choctaw heritage.

However, Indigenous peoples are often held to a level of distinction and cultural continuity not demanded of others, so that when Choctaws are called upon to "be Choctaw," to be "authentic," to perform authenticity (Barker 2011; Cattelino 2010; Dennison 2012; Povinelli 2002)—that is, an authentic Choctaw identity, an authentic Choctaw heritage, a heritage that must render Choctaws distinctive as both individuals and as a collective—for many, it is impossible. It is an impossible performance of authenticity that aligns with or participates in the authorized heritage discourse to present "authentic" (i.e., acceptable) ideas of Indianness such as stickball, dancing, and other traditional cultural expressions. Within the authorized heritage discourse, certain kinds of heritage serve as identifiers for authenticity among Indigenous peoples—*authentic* Indianness. These include ideas of traditional cultural expressions such as language, dresses, stickball, and so on. For example, one woman shared how her grandfather, a "full-blood" Choctaw, wears a headdress (she called it a "Native costume") to her daughter's school during Thanksgiving.

> At Thanksgiving, he's gone to my girl's school every year dressed up in his Native costume, headdress and, like, a Choctaw shirt. I talk about him. Every year I talk about him. It's like the story gets a little bit more, because I find out more information, because I'll say, "Well, tell me about this," or whatever. I did find out that his mom was born here but his grandparents walked the Trail of Tears here, from Mississippi." (Annie, McAlester)

Striking is the complexity of Annie's grandfather's Indianness: He couples a headdress—which is not traditional to Choctaws, but widely recognized as "authentically" Indian in mainstream American culture—with a Choctaw shirt, recognized as "authentically" Indian, but only to those who know what a Choctaw shirt looks like. His grandparents walked the Trail of Tears, an *authentic* Indian experience, but he doesn't offer this information easily, as his granddaughter, a middle-aged women, has only just now discovered this; she learns more about him and the rest of her family when he gives public talks *to others*. Thus, there is a performativity of Indianness that actively falls within the authorized heritage discourse at the individual level and another type of indigeneity (a "Choctawness") that is not recognized within the authorized heritage discourse.

Tribal citizens may link their individual and collective identities with heritage in multiple ways: actively or passively within the authorized heritage discourse; in active opposition to the authorized heritage discourse; or without reference to any of it at all. The tribe, however, links Choctaw identity with heritage actively within the authorized heritage discourse. This active linkage is visible in multiple forms, including the presentations of traditional cultural expressions already described, but also in other interesting ways. For example, in travel plazas across the reservation, the tribe sells a number of Native-inspired memorabilia including beaded moccasins, dream catchers, beaded jewelry, t-shirts, keychains, mugs, etc., presumably for the many tourists traveling to the area seeking "authentic" Indian souvenirs. What is particularly interesting about these objects, however, is that they are manufactured in China and play into circulating notions about what being Indian is *supposed* to mean (to non-Indians), and further, how Indians *fit* into the larger mainstream American narrative.[8] Avoiding the tangled intricacies of who is performing

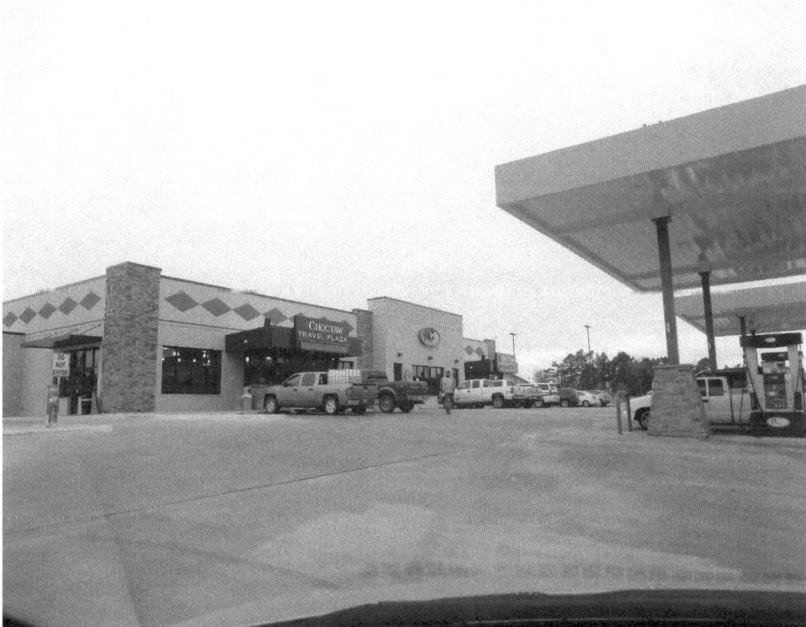

FIGURE 9 Choctaw Nation Travel Plaza, Antlers, Oklahoma. Note the Choctaw diamond pattern that decorates the top of the building. Photo by Kasey Jernigan (author).

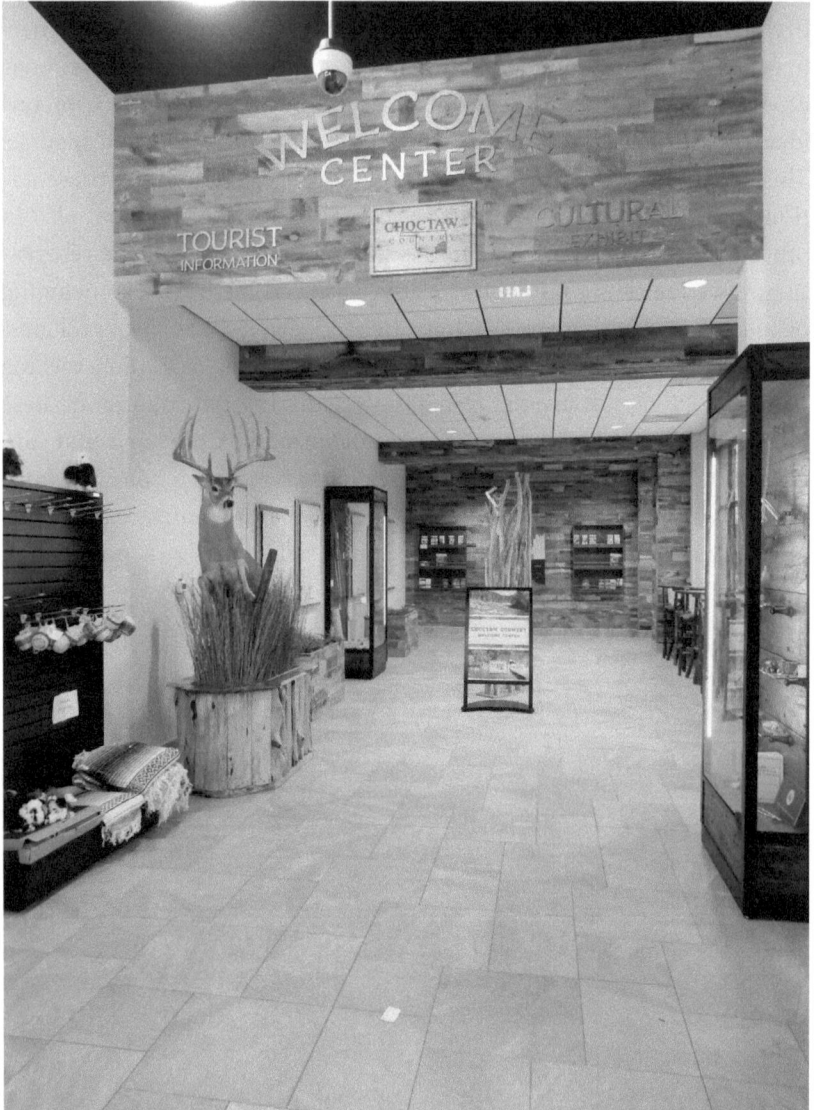

FIGURE 10 Welcome Center/Museum inside Travel Plaza, Antlers, Oklahoma. This Welcome Center/Museum offers material culture and informational boards on Choctaw cultural traditions such as storytelling, dancing, and origin stories. Photo by Kasey Jernigan (author).

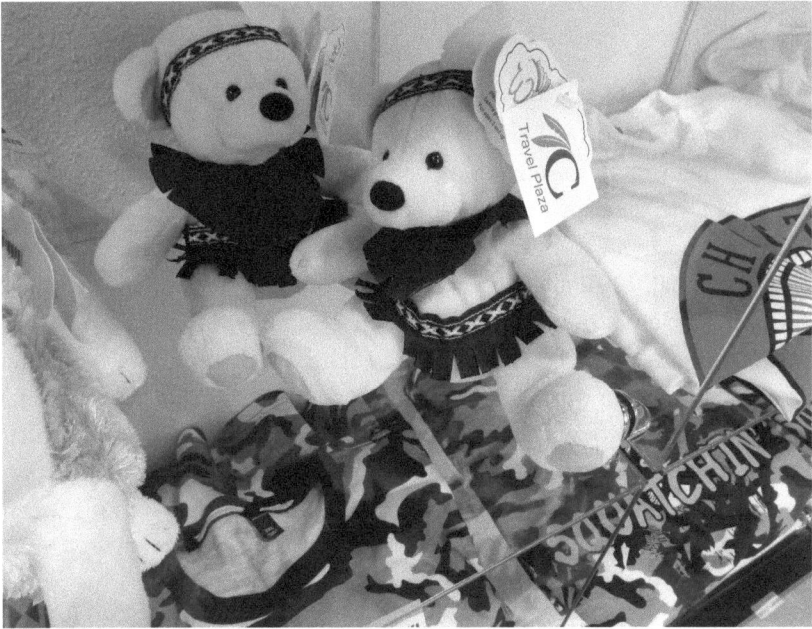

FIGURE 11 Teddy bears dressed as Indians sold at the Travel Plaza, Antlers, Oklahoma. Photo by Kasey Jernigan (author).

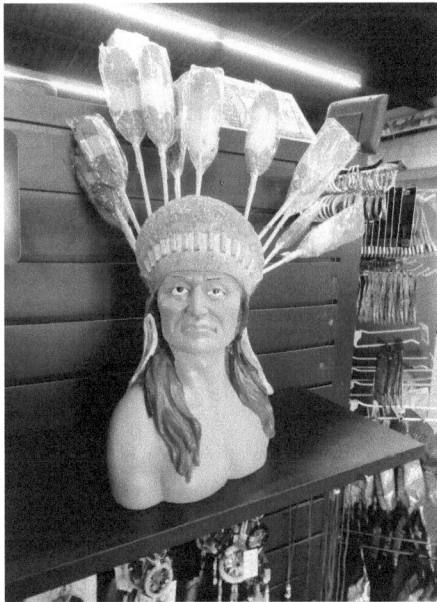

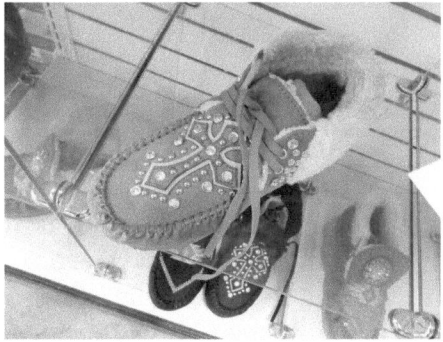

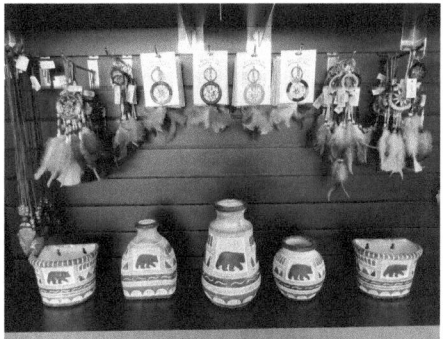

FIGURE 12 Items for sale at the Travel Plaza, Durant, Oklahoma. Photos by Kasey Jernigan (author).

for whom (and for what purpose), Smith (2012) argues that tourists are not mere observers of heritage performances (authentic or otherwise) but are themselves performers whose actions do cultural work. Moreover, it is the tourists' meaning-making and values brought with them (or inspiring them to purchase these goods) where authenticity can be found. Bagnall (2015:88) describes an emotional authenticity in which tourist engagement with heritage produces an emotional response that is "meaningful and real." Smith (2012:215) argues that tourists' moments of performance "may be shallow, banal and simply focused on entertainment; others may be profound, deep and emotionally resonant, in which something is perhaps "learned," newly understood or re-worked. However, they will be active, and they will be *authentic*—by which I mean they will have real contemporary cultural meaning, of whatever significance, to the performer of that moment.

During my time in the field, in 2016, there was a quite a bit of talk among the women that Oklahoma was considering changing legislation to allow casinos to open and operate across the state, not just on Indian lands. One woman described how she had just come from a meeting with tribal council members in Durant, and the tribe was purchasing land in Hochatown, the top tourist destination in the Choctaw Nation. The plan was to build a waterpark and family cabins to cater to the tourists from Dallas who come up for lake holidays. She commented that there was a sense of panic that new non-tribal casinos would take away revenue from the tribe, so the Nation was planning to diversify its investments.[9] I was struck by the sense of panic she described and began thinking about it in terms of heritage and the tribe's newly energized efforts to put forth a distinct (and "authentic") Choctaw identity, to make their travel plazas and casino resorts a distinct (and "authentic") Choctaw experience. Is there is too much at stake to be "adaptable" now, or perhaps this is in the spirit of adaptability?

Heritage carries power as a legitimizing or delegitimizing discourse (Smith 2006), and moreover, heritage has a political power that rests within its naturalization as material object. Thus, the merchandise the tribe sells is material heritage; they are objects symbolic of not only identities, but also of certain values. As Smith (2006:53) notes, "Heritage may be embodied as objects of desire and prestige in and of themselves, not because of any inherent value, but in so far as the symbolic ability to control desired, fetishized and prized objects reinforces not only the identity, but the power of the identity of the nation, group or individual in possession." The tribe, through selling "Made in China" Indian heritage (merchandise), participates in a bizarre process within the authorized heritage discourse in which Choctaws are at once legitimized, fetishized, and corporatized as "Indians." This does not occur unseen, and for some, this linkage of heritage and identity within the authorized heritage discourse leads to feelings of confusion and distrust. One woman described this so eloquently:

> What is our culture? What is the real culture? And that's what I'm saying. You going back from our ancestors or from now? So, see, that's what's hard for me to get. Where are we at? Because our ancestors was in Mississippi. Well, then, see, we didn't come from Mississippi. We come from Oklahoma. Maybe our great grandma and them was, but see, when we get over here that tradition over there is Mississippi tradition. So that's why I say I can't really get, you know, what's the right culture? And that's why it's hard for me to make someone understand how I feel, because I don't know which one's real. I mean, which one you should go with, you know?

These ideas of an "authentic Indianness" come undone in the day-to-day. They come undone in the banal, everyday processes of "just being together" and just being Choctaw, outside of an authorized heritage discourse. As such, it appears that there is something like a counter-authenticity, a counter-heritage[10] that *is* the banal or the everyday, lived, and embodied heritage-making around, for example, "just being together" and eating food together. Furthermore, when heritage includes struggle and hardship related to loss of land, foodways, language, and traditions—the non-aesthetically pleasing histories—this is not recognized within the authorized heritage discourse. But Indigenous people creatively engage with these demands for authenticity (Barker 2011; Cattelino 2010; Dennison 2012; Povinelli 2002). Foods, foodways, and fat bodies are one such example of how Indigenous peoples reconcile the past in the present: Large bodies give shape and meaning to one aspect of their identity (Jernigan 2013; Vantrese 2013). As Darla, a woman from my exploratory fieldwork noted, fat bodies work as social connectors and markers of Indianness.

Conclusion

This chapter opened with an account of the Trail of Tears Commemorative Walk to illustrate that the commemoration itself is an act of heritage that includes passing on knowledge (through storytelling), engaging with remembering, embodiment (i.e., physically walking), bringing together people for a sense of community in a place that symbolizes historical and cultural values and meanings. Thus, it was everything happening during the commemorative walk, and at the chosen sites, that made it heritage, not the mere fact of the annual walk's existence. Indeed, that is what heritage is: not a "thing," but a cultural process.

The authorized heritage discourse is the dominant view of heritage that privileges expert values over those of community and local interests and which works to constrain understandings of heritage as primarily material. The field of critical heritage studies, and Laurajane Smith (2006) in particular, has challenged the authorized heritage discourse to reframe heritage as a cultural process that engages with acts of remembering, which work to create ways to understand and engage with the present. The embodied heritage framework utilizes Smith's conceptualization of heritage as the "process of remembering that underpins identity and the ways in which individuals and groups make sense of their experiences in the present," and in this chapter, I offer examples from women's heritage narratives that link heritage with identity, Indigenous relationality, and meaning-making.

Women's narratives highlight the ways in which heritage is used to describe traditional cultural expressions, such as *Chahta anumpa*, clothing, stickball, and more. These notions of cultural heritage are evoked as a way to focus on solidarity and cultural continuity among Choctaws. This is indeed what happens; there is solidarity and cultural continuity in maintaining these practices, and they serve as tools that help to remember the past, make sense of the present, and shape identities (Smith 2006, 2007). Yet, as this research shows, these traditional cultural expressions become reified in particular ways, especially in the context of identity-making and legitimization. Indigenous peoples are often held to a level of distinction not demanded of others, and for Choctaws, many of whom do not participate in cultural expressions that render them "authentic" or distinct, this demand is impossible to live up to. It is a demand that works to erase what it really means to be Choctaw. Thus, the authorized heritage discourse comes in handy as a way to respond to demands for authenticity, and the tribe at large utilizes the authorized heritage discourse to actively link heritage and tribal identity.

Throughout women's narratives, references to historical trauma appear and are framed as dissonant heritage as a way to understand how women process, cope with, and make sense of ambivalent and traumatic pasts. Choctaws often call on past struggle from historical trauma to define qualities of resiliency and adaptability that they use in the present in response to contemporary forms of violence and inequality. But also, these memories serve as a way to demand more from themselves and to hold themselves accountable to do their very best within the constraints in which they live.

CHAPTER 5

Food, Foodways, Identity, Belonging, and Obesity

I met Jessica at the Food Distribution market in Durant, the headquarters of the Choctaw Nation. In June 2014, the Durant market was the first of five stores the tribe opened. It is a two-million-dollar, 7,500-square-foot center designed to feel like a small grocery store. At the ribbon cutting ceremony, Minko Batton stated:

> Years ago we used to deliver our food out in trucks. Our people had to line up in their vehicles and had to wait until the food was delivered to them. So it was really a humiliating time for them. This allows them to have honor, dignity . . . all are welcome to make multiple trips to any of the centers during business hours, and a weekly trip—[as] opposed to monthly—will use less storage space and allow clients to keep their supply fresh. (Trista Winnett, store manager for the Durant location, personal communication 2014)

Jessica was at the Durant market to pick up her family's food for the month of March. While the idea of a weekly trip to the Food Distribution store was appealing, it just wasn't feasible for her or for many of the families living within the boundaries of the Choctaw Nation. Jessica lives in a tiny, rural town with a population of approximately two hundred people, nearly an hour away from the Durant store. At the time we met, she was twenty-three years old, living in a two-bedroom, multi-generational house that she shared with her boyfriend, her mother, her fourteen-year-old brother, eighteen-year-old sister, and her great-grandmother, for whom Jessica was the full-time caregiver. Their home was located on a single dirt road, just off the town's main street, and was one of a handful of homes surrounded by the remnants of attrition: rusty broken-down cars, tires, and discarded sheet metal. Were there not a pack of dogs chasing my car, I would have mistaken the street for abandoned, forgotten at minimum. Jessica's house was a bit down the dirt road, just past a bubbling creek that had a couple of drywall boards tossed over it as a make-shift bridge. I drove slowly over the haphazardly improvised bridge—fearing the "bridge" would break from the weight of my car—and nearly passed their house. None of the dwellings had numbers or signage, but a young man, whom I found out later was Jessica's boyfriend, was sitting outside on the porch and waved me down while hollering over his shoulder to someone inside.

I pulled into their yard where he gestured, parked on the wet grass, and got out of the car. The huddle of small dogs that had been chasing the car rushed to surround my legs, jumping, nipping, and barking. Jessica's house was one of the nicer homes, as indicated by its solid roof and structurally sound appearance. Smiling warmly, she rushed out to meet me. Her energy was generous and welcoming yet busy and scattered as she waved me inside. Jessica was cooking breakfast and had just begun to plate food for her family members, who were sitting on brown velour-patterned couches, watching television in the adjacent room. As I entered their home, the heavy, stagnant smell of cooked sausage and cramped conditions marbled the air.

It would be too simple to describe their home as cluttered, as that fails to capture the effect of poverty—crowded spaces, a worlding of generational belongings, stories, memories, and experiences of lives compromised, made and unmade over and over, in this shelter, their home. A short shelf of collectable dolls was displayed prominently against the wall, three dozen or so assorted dolls dressed as "Hollywood Indians" with buckskin clothing, feathers, beads, braids, some with bright glassy brown eyes wide open—all collected across generations. Stacks of newspapers, boxes, odd vintage furniture, and plastic decorations filled the entry, which opened directly into their dining room/kitchen. After everyone was settled with their food, Jessica and I sat at the small circular dining table, nearly fully covered with items that had nowhere else to go, and began our conversation.

Jessica's narrative had all the harbingers of Billy-Ray Belcourt's (2018:2) exhausted existence of indigeneity, "the miserable feeling of not properly being of this world." As we talked, she shared story after story with me: her personal experiences of physical, sexual, and emotional abuse; failed relationships; mental health struggles and a suicide attempt that she recognized as her "rock bottom." She motioned repeatedly to her body as she spoke, unable to hide the disgust and shame she carries for her own fat, diseased body. I was once again reminded of Belcourt's claim that "colonial affects escape analytic capture," once again moved by how easy it truly would be to think that the reservation "is bad for life because its members are bad at life" (2018:1–2). During our visit, she shared with me her family's personal histories and intergenerational traumas of disenfranchisement, children forced to attend Indian boarding schools, material and cultural dispossession, and shaken onto-epistemologies. Depending on the government for food—more specifically, as Jessica described it, for "fatty, starchy, high-calorie, preserved commodity foods that give us all commod bods"—was just another feature of these interconnected experiences. And it was here in this statement that I recognized how Jessica (and so many others in this project) utilizes the framework of historical trauma as public narrative to make sense of contemporary health disparities.

In this chapter, I bring together concepts of food, identity, and belonging found across women's food-centered life stories to examine the associations of fat bodies and Indianness in the lives of Choctaw women, offering a window into the ways in which they understand disease as a manifestation of this "exhausted existence of indigeneity—of not properly being of this world." I begin by presenting cultural and traditional foods and foodways as described by women in the Choctaw Nation, followed by the ways they link these with fatness. Next, I examine the Food Distribution Program (FDP) at a local level and describe an everyday shopping experience at one store, followed by women's accounts of their FDP experiences. Then, I offer women's understandings of obesity and related conditions (e.g., diabetes) and the ways they make sense of these experiences; how their meaning-making works to politicize biology, re-

vealing the intersections where sick (Indigenous) bodies are simultaneously produced, surveilled, and governed, and where obesity manifests as
a racialized symptom of a world hijacked and constructed on the settler
notion that Indigenous peoples were (and are) always-already dying off
(Belcourt 2018). In doing so, I demonstrate which social forces are at
the heart of the embodied heritage framework and discuss the broader
implications of embodied heritage apart from obesity.

Foods and Foodways

"Eating together lies at the heart of social relations; at meals we create
family and friendships by sharing food, tastes, values, and ourselves"
(Counihan 1999:6). Food is central to both biological and social life, and
meals mark celebrations and enlarge the social group across events such
as church dinners, potlucks, and kinship celebrations. Food is endlessly
meaningful, its significance boundless; food is a product and reflection
of social organization at the broadest and most intimate levels (Counihan 1999; Douglas 1966). An examination of foodways—behaviors and
beliefs surrounding the production, distribution, and consumption of
food—reveals much about relations of power, the intersection of gender
roles, and familial and societal structures, as well as the intricate fabric
of meanings, symbols, and language. Because of our fundamental, daily
need for food, "food was, and continues to be, power in a most basic, tangible and inescapable form" (Arnold 1988:3), and eating together, sharing
food collectively, is a sign of kinship, trust, and friendship, which is crucial to the very definition of community and relationships between people (Mauss 1967:58). In other words, the act of eating with others signifies
close bonds, trust, and relating, which are essential to community and
human connections. The core message here is clear: Eating is not merely
a biological need but a social act that binds humans (and non-humans)
to each other and to place; and food is central to creating and nurturing
a collective identity and sense of belonging.

Intimately related to the local environment, foods and foodways influence the shaping of community, family, and memories—people articulate and recognize their collective distinctiveness through the medium of
food (Bell and Valentine 1997; Brown and Mussell 1984; Counihan 1999;

Williams et al 2012). Foodways offer a window to understanding a people's history, values, social structures, and relationships with space and place. Food's role in shaping identity and culture is profound; it anchors us to our pasts, narrates our present, and seeds our futures, all at the same time. Food is an inherently visceral experience that has the capacity to connect the eaters to the vast narratives of their cultures, ensuring that their practices, stories, and very essence are continually nourished and kept alive, providing an important platform for people to (re)affirm their identities and develop social bonds.

I want to emphasize again that I use the term *identity* carefully, acknowledging that the word itself lacks the complexity of relationality. As Kim TallBear reminds us, "[I]dentity . . . does not necessarily imply ongoing relating. It exist[s] as a largely individualistic idea, as something considered to be held once and for all unchanging within one's body. Whether through biological or social imprinting, identity is often considered as one's body's property" (2019). Language choice is powerful, and like food, it shapes and reflects understanding. I hope to use the term *identity* with more precision and intent, to ensure that the collective nature of Choctaw relationality is not obscured by narrower interpretations of *identity* as a mere individual trait or choice—the goal being to highlight *not* a strictly personal dimension of identity, but rather the nexus of our experiences, concerns, stories, ways of knowing and being as situated in relationality. In other words, in what ways do foods, foodways, and eating serve as conduits for identity-making and belonging (through kinship, collectivity, or other communal bonds) among Choctaws? It's about the collective narrative more than a solitary one; it's a focus not on the lens of personal identity, but rather a deeper collective significance that includes relating with humans and non-humans as well (TallBear 2019).

For southeastern tribes (i.e., the Choctaw, Chickasaw, Cherokee, and Creek), traditional foods and agricultural practices are embodiments of their relationship with the land, ancestors, and community. Known as skilled farmers, these tribes traditionally subsisted on about 60 percent agriculture and 40 percent hunting and gathering (Intertribal Agriculture Council 2018). Few tribes around the country relied so heavily on agriculture, and several modern farming techniques are thought to have originated with them. Corn, beans, and squash, the clever companion-planting system dubbed the "three sisters," are more than nutrient-rich staples to these cultures; they represent centuries of farming wisdom and a deep respect for the land's gifts. Jessica described for me how she learned of the three sisters: "The corn is like the tall sister, shooting up towards the sky. The beans climb up with a little support and wind around the stalks, like an ever-reaching middle child. And the squash grows low on the ground and covers it, keeping weeds from growing, like the fat, lazy sister!"

Upon forced removal to Indian Territory, Choctaws continued with agriculture, getting to know the new lands in southeastern Oklahoma. Today, agriculture and gardening remain an important part of life, and the women I spoke with each had her own tale of tending to family gardens as a child: days spent stooping alongside rows of greens, fingers buried in the soil of small gardens or larger farmlands. Today, many of these women have smaller personal gardens, but the number who actively cultivate them has dwindled. The obstacles they face are many—extreme weather that brings scorching heat, torrential rains and floods, and tornado season which has now expanded beyond just the spring; the demands of hectic schedules, including driving across the rural counties to transport family to events or to run errands like food shopping; and many are also held back by health issues such as obesity, diabetes, and other chronic conditions. But even those who've never planted a seed as adults were adamant that they could cultivate a garden if they tried: They feel connected to these agricultural foodways through their memories, experiences, and the sense that these ways of knowing and being are ingrained in who they are and how they relate with the living landscape.

Those who do continue to grow their own foods described with deep affection how their garden tomatoes blush red on the vine, spicy peppers and crisp cucumbers grow boldly, and their joy when the distinct pods of okra first sprout from the soil in their gardens. None of it goes to waste. The harvests are used in home-cooked meals, generously shared with neighbors and friends, or preserved in jars for later use. What's more, these foods also offer opportunities to create cherished bonds with others across time and space. Women recalled vivid memories of plucking peaches and snapping beans with loved ones, as most of their food memories are associated with parents, aunties, uncles, and grandparents. These are also experiences they recreate with their own children, grandchildren, and other young people, including how to care for excess foods and prepare for the changing season. They recalled learning how to can and preserve the peaches, beans, and other grown foods, and those who garden today do so with a responsibility in mind: to pass on memories and teachings to their children and grandchildren, aware that the world is still being made, it is still in formation, and they have roles and responsibilities in this yet-incomplete worlding.

Growing food to feed one's family is a social process that produces food, brings people together, and builds relations with the plants and lands. One of my favorite parts of this project was talking with women about these food memories. They relished the opportunity to remember and share these moments, smiling, laughing, crying, transporting us momentarily to a time and place that felt as real and meaningful as the conversation we were having in the moment. I recall, for example, how Wilma, an elder from Broken Bow who became an auntie to me, wanting to teach me *Chahta anumpa* and teasing me like only an auntie can, smiled and lit up when she talked about a food memory.

> My family planting the gardens, and we were just—when we were picking, we would be eating it, whatever it was! If it was onions or tomatoes, whatever it was, we were picking this stuff out of the garden and we was eating it! We didn't care, we didn't wash it, we'd just eat it! And that right there is my fondest memory of food as a child and being with my family, my grandparents, and my parents, everybody getting together to do the gardening, the big gardens. Because they canned it, we canned it; we put up our own food and if we had that, we really, we was millionaires! I haven't [gardened] in many years. My husband got sick and after he got sick, we kind of slacked for many, many years, and now we haven't been able, but we used to. I used to can and taught the grandkids, the boys, to can all kinds of things and make jelly and everything.

These women have lived their entire lives in a world that has been rapidly changing. They have witnessed and been part of the changing foodways, and they echoed a common sentiment—that it's not just the unrivaled taste of home-grown, freshly picked produce from one's garden at stake, but also the erosion of relationality, of heritage, of ways of knowing and being that have long been nourished by the practices of growing one's own food. I heard story after story of women lamenting these losses, and the ways they talked about these experiences, comparing them to their lives now, underscored the absence of these practices and all that is associated with them. They described sitting outside, peeling fruits, preparing them for canning, surrounded by aunties and grandmas—experiences that were about more than just preserving food. This is where family came together: Each family would take home a share, but it was the unity, the shared efforts, the stories, teasing, joking, learning, the "just being together" that truly "fed" them.

Many of the women in this project believe that convenience has affected how they relate to foods and each other (even as they complained about how inconvenient it can be to get groceries). Some reminisced about their youth, when going to a food store required a ten-mile trek, often in harsh conditions—this labor notably less enjoyable than the labor of "foodwork" with family. They described walking in blazing hot heat or through "sticker patches" to get to the nearest store where they could charge a few grocery items. They associate the convenience of store-bought foods and the decline in gardening among young people with increasing health issues within the Choctaw Nation. The women recalled a time when health problems like obesity and diabetes were rare and attribute this to the active lifestyle demanded at the time, as well as the organic, locally sourced diets that were simply the most accessible foodways of their youth. As foodways have changed in their lifetimes, so too has life expectancy, it seems to them. I heard multiple stories about how their elders lived very long lives and were rarely sick. Diabetes was unheard of. Whereas today, American Indians have the lowest life expectancy among any population in the United States. Moreover, the irony of the contemporary (healthy) move toward organic food is not lost on them: Organic, locally grown foods are a return to how they grew up eating, but these foods are no longer affordable or easily accessible where they live; instead, they have come to be associated with whiteness and wealth.

In addition to gardening, other Choctaw foodways remain relevant today, some argue in part because of the rurality of their locations. They hunt, fish the many waterways, and forage for local wildlife and plants, supplemented by wild berries, pokeweed, wild onions, and various "field greens" like dandelion and lamb's-quarter. These are considered important, necessary, and meaningful cultural foodways. Hunting is generally thought of as mostly men's work, but everyone takes pride in (and is a part of) these specific food-getting methods that have always been central to Choctaw foodways. Deer is the primary game hunted today (with squirrels and rabbits not as common as during these women's childhoods) and is often generously shared with families, friends, and neighbors. Recall Carmen from the previous chapter, whose husband is well known for hunting deer and sharing it with others. She explained that they hunt in the rural woods where deer roam unobstructed and consume local plants grown organically and in relation with their surroundings. She described how her husband considers himself vegetarian because when he consumes the deer, he is consuming the vegetation that sustained the deer. The deer is not separate from its surroundings and is alive only because of the plants and larger ecosystems that sustain it.

While these food-getting activities are a cherished part of their cultural heritage, the women acknowledged the challenges they face in sustaining these practices, such as obtaining hunting licenses, the physical demands involved, and the laborious steps of washing, processing, and cooking the food. But despite the difficulties, these foodways remain a meaningful and necessary aspect of their way of life, and they are taken very seriously. For example, spring marks the beginning of wild onion season, and women have sacred, special places where they pick wild onions. Wild onions, a seasonal and hard-to-find edible, are treasured, often cooked with eggs, and are a special treat. Spring—wild onion season—also marks the start of fundraising, dinners at churches or cultural centers where volunteers cook wild onions, eggs, salt pork, and fry bread, selling plates for about nine dollars. In urban centers like *Tvlse* (Tulsa), it is common to find Indigenous peoples from multiple tribes gathering to enjoy wild onion dinners. They are revered and celebrated. Therefore, possessing the knowledge of where to harvest wild onions is highly valued and can also be quite lucrative. Some families are known to guard the location of their onion patches closely, and each year they gather, prepare, and sell them, sometimes for a hefty sum. My grandmother used to tell the story of being pregnant with my dad and, while picking wild onions with her sister, went into labor. She and Annie stopped picking the wild onions and prioritized relocating to a space that was more widely known so as to protect their secret wild onion patch. They were concerned about protecting and keeping safe the "where" of the wild onion spot they had found and would (re)visit for years and years with their own children and grandchildren. These spots and the knowledge of where to find wild onions, how to pick them, clean them, and cook them, is passed down through generations. Because of the severity and success of assimilation, these knowledges are often forgone. Yet, wild onions continue to grow.

Food Distribution Program

The tribe currently has five Food Distribution locations across its ten-and-a-half counties. For this project, I visited four stores—McAlester, Durant, Broken Bow, and Poteau—selected for their wide distribution across the reservation boundaries. The Choctaw Nation has invested deeply in the Food Distribution stores. Costing an estimated $2 million each to complete, the stores are designed to mimic a typical grocery-store shopping experience, including aisles of foods to choose from, a fresh produce stand, and refrigerators containing vegetables, cheese, and meats. At the Durant store's opening ceremony, Jerry Tonubbee, the Food Distribution Program director, noted, "It's almost like being at Wal-Mart or any other small grocery store. You come in, get your food, and go through our scanners. Then we scan it out. The only difference is you don't give us any money." Minko Batton added, "This is one of many things we're going to do. There's this [store]; we're going to do one in the McAlester area; we're going to do one in the Broken Bow area. But it's because we finally have the funds to make things like this happen." Mr. Tonubbee and the staff at the Food Distribution stores frequently commented on the benefits of this new grocery-store style market, de-scribing that people can come and go as they please and as often as they want, rather than having to get all their food at once (Trista Winnett, store manager for the Durant location, personal communication 2014).

Low-income households living within the boundaries of the Nation that contain at least one person who is a member of a federally recog-nized tribe are eligible to participate in the Food Distribution Program on Indian Reservations (FDPIR). Households are certified based on fi-nancial (e.g., income) and non-financial standards set by the federal gov-ernment and must be recertified at least every twelve months.[1] To sign up for the FDPIR, a face-to-face meeting with a staff member is required. To arrange this, one must first consult the FDPIR's monthly schedule via the FDPIR calendar, which is printed in the *Biskinik*, the monthly Choctaw Nation newspaper, as well as on the Choctaw Nation's website. Once a potential new client has determined the best date to come in for the required interview, they must bring copies of their 1) Certificate of Degree of Indian Blood (CDIB) card or tribal membership card—their file must contain proof of tribal lineage; 2) Social Security cards for all household members; 3) proof of address; 4) income verification—this takes the form of the last four paystubs; verification of Social Security or Department of Health Services (DHS) stipends for fixed-income clients; for those unemployed, proof of registration with the unemployment office or collateral statements of unemployment from two non-relatives; or for students, copies of tuition, books and fees, and verification of grants and loans received; and 5) a termination letter from the DHS for those who applied for or received SNAP (food stamp) benefits. The Food Distribution stores are open Monday through Wednesday and Fridays, 8:00 a.m. to 4:30 p.m., and Thursdays from 9:00 a.m. to 5:30 p.m. They are closed the last two days of the month for inventory, as well as federal and tribal holidays (which include the birthdays of tribal council members).

Inside each store is a small sitting area, usually just to the right of the entry, where potential clients can sit and wait to be seen. At my visit to the Durant store, there were several televisions overhead, one running a presentation of nutritional education (e.g., how much sugar is in common foods and drinks) on a loop; another was running a healthy cooking show (*Kids a Cookin' with Karen*). Karen, a white nutritionist at Kansas State University, was teaching a young boy how to make peachy pork picante and pasta salad.[2] Just behind the seats, on the wall, was a framed picture of the Ten Commandments, in English on the left and *Chahta anumpa* on the right. Below the Ten Commandments was an open shelf with dozens of pamphlets offering advice, tips, and information on, for example, "Workday Fitness: Let's Get Moving," or "25 Ways to Support Walking and Bicycling in Our Community," "Home Energy Audits from the Choctaw Nation Housing Authority," and a Choctaw healthy eating calendar.

Once determined eligible and approved, shoppers (or clients, as they're often referred to) can get a shopping cart or motorized wheelchair with a basket attached and a household shopping list (i.e., a check sheet) that offers an inventoried list of items, broken down by category, and the allowed pounds per category. Household shopping lists are available for households ranging from one person to twelve people. Each person in a household is allowed approximately eighty-five pounds of food per month, broken down as follows: eleven pounds of vegetables; ten pounds of fruit; four pounds of canned and dried beans; five pounds of pasta and rice; as well as—not categorized by pounds—two bottles of juice; two egg mixes; three meat items; one peanut product; one fats product (butter or vegetable oil); four cans of evaporated milk and one instant milk or four UHT milks[3] (but those two options must be alternated each month); one hot cereal; one cheese option, every other month; two flour and cornmeal containers; one box dried cereal; one bakery mix, every four months; three canned soups; and one box of crackers. There are multiple substitution options; some items are available only every other month, or you must alternate with other items each month. Some foods count differently: For example, russet potatoes count as "five pounds" and red potatoes count as "three pounds." See the shopping list in Figure 13 for an example for a household of four.

If this sounds confusing, it is. We might consider Strakosch's (2024:24) analysis of policy and bureaucracy helpful for understanding the confusion and violence of neoliberal colonial bureaucracy, whereby "bureaucracy is an organisational form structuring all contemporary policy systems in neoliberal settler colonies. While many point to the problems that beset policymaking in Indigenous affairs—hierarchical decision-making, paternalism, the problematisation of Indigenous lives and so on—we rarely connect these problems to the underlying bureaucratic structure that conditions them. . . . It is useful to think of bureaucracy as producing a particular interventionist state orientation to Indigenous worlds, allowing the state to enact colonial violence while framing it as technical best practice and, ultimately, as a form of care."

The Nation designed, planned, and built the Food Distribution stores to mimic grocery stores, offering what Minko Batton described as a more honorable and dignified approach to obtaining government-supplied foods, yet the experiences I observed seem more aptly described as sites of contested struggle related to sovereignty (Strakosch 2024). The tribe harnesses the Food Distribution Program on Indian Reservations (FDPIR) to fulfill its inherent duty of caring for its citizens and lands, en-

HOUSEHOLD OF 4 SHOPPING LIST   NAME: _____

VEGETABLES
ALLOWED 44 POUNDS OF VEGETABLES **MAY SUBSTITUTE UP TO 20 POUNDS OF FRUIT FOR VEGETABLES**
___1# KERNAL CORN
___1# TOMATOES
___1# HOMINY
___1# MIXED VEGETABLES
___1# GREEN BEANS
___1# CARROTS
___1# CREAM CORN
___1# PUMPKIN
___1#PEAS
___1# SPINACH

___1# SLICED POTATOES
___1# BAG INSTANT POTATOES
___1# SPAGHETTI SAUCE
___1# TOMATO SAUCE
___1# CARROTS
___1# YELLOW ONIONS
___5# RUSSETT POTATOES
___3# RED POTATOES
___1# SOUP MIX
___1# FRESH SWEET POTATOES
___1# FRESH CABBAGE
___1# PURPLE ONION
___1# BELL PEPPERS
___1# CELERY
___1# TOMATOES
___1# ROMAINE LETTUCE
___1# FRESH CAULIFLOWER
___1# BROCCOLI
___1# RADISHES

FRUIT
ALLOWED 40 POUNDS OF FRUIT **MAY SUBSTITUTE UP TO 20 POUNDS OF FRUIT FOR VEGETABLES**
___1# APPLESAUCE
___1# APRICOTS
___1# FRUIT COCKTAIL
___1# PEACHES

___1# PEARS

___1# BAG OF PRUNES
___1# BOX OF RAISINS
___3# RED APPLES
___3# GRANNY SMITH APPLES
___5# GRAPEFRUIT
___5# ORANGES
___5# MIXED FRUIT

JUICE
ALLOWED 8 BOTTLES
___GRAPE
___TOMATO
___ORANGE
___GRAPEFRUIT
___CRANAPPLE
___APPLE

CANNED & DRY BEANS
ALLOWED 16 POUNDS
___1# CANNED PINTO BEANS
___1# CANNED BLACK BEANS
___1# CANNED KIDNEY BEANS
___1#CANNED VEGETARIAN BEANS
___1# CANNED REFRIED BEANS
___2# DRY PINTO BEANS
___2# DRY GREAT NORTHERN

EGG MIX
___ALLOWED 8

MEATS
ALLOWED 12 ITEMS
___FROZEN WHOLE CHICKEN
___FRZ GROUND BEEF (2-1)
___FROZEN BEEF ROAST
___CANNED BEEF
___SALMON (2-1)
___FROZEN CHICKEN BREAST
___CANNED CHICKEN (2-1)
___PORK CHOPS (2-1)

PEANUT PRODUCTS
ALLOWED 4
___PEANUT BUTTER
___PEANUTS
___FRUIT & NUT MIX

FATS
___6 BUTTERY SPREAD OR
___2 REAL BUTTER OR
___2 VEGETABLE OIL
(SEE CLERK FOR MORE OPTIONS)

MILK
___EVAP. MILK –16 CANS

INSTANT AND UHT MILK
CHOOSE 1 OPTION
___2 INSTANT MILK
___16 UHT MILK
___1 INSTANT AND 8 UHT MILK

HOT CEREAL
ALLOWED 4
___FARINA
___OATMEAL

CHEESE
ALLOWED 2
___SLICED
___BLOCK

PASTA & RICE
ALLOWED 20 POUNDS
___1# WH. GRAIN ROTINI
___1# EGG NOODLES
___1# MACARONI &

CHEESE (ALLOWED 3 PER PERSON IN HH)
___2# RICE
___1# SPAGHETTI

FLOUR & CORNMEAL
ALLOWED 8
___CORNMEAL
___FLOUR
___WHOLE WHEAT FLOUR

DRY CEREAL
ALLOWED 4 BOXES
___CORN & RICE
___WHEAT BRAN
___OAT CIRCLES
___CORN SQUARE
___RICE CRISP
___CORN FLAKES

BAKERY MIX
___ALLOWED 1

CANNED SOUPS
ALLOWED 12
___VEGETABLE SOUP
___TOMATO SOUP
___CHUNKY BEEF STEW
___CREAM OF CHICKEN SOUP
___CREAM OF MUSROOM SOUP

CRACKERS
___ALLOWED 4

FIGURE 13 Household of four's shopping list. Reproduced by Kasey Jernigan (author).

acting political power not through overt lobbying or direct interactions with the federal government (though this does happen) but at a more fundamental level of control and governance rooted in Choctaw social responsibility. Maneuvering within federal policy frameworks, the tribe's grocery-store style FDPIR shops were constructed with tribal citizens in mind. That is, the tribe continues to care for its citizens—and particularly their humanity—with methods deeply intertwined with "the long past and necessary future of Indigenous sovereignties," (Strakosch 2024:21) but also within state-authorized policy frameworks.

Minko Batton claims that these stores allow for a more dignified way to collect one's commodity foods. I argue that while that may be true, what is more interesting to me is how Choctaw sovereignty is contested in these sites. Specifically, how "dignity" and "honor" are used as a register of care (and for whom) when the experience of being Indigenous and depending on commodity foods is anything but dignified or honorable. First, "clients" do not come and go as they please, picking up, for example, fresh meat to cook for dinner the same night. The towns in which people live are rural (hence the need for the FDPIR in lieu of SNAP), and although the tribal campuses (which house the FDPIR stores, wellness centers, Head Start schools, and community centers) have aimed to be in the centers of the counties, many are a long drive away for most people. The tribe does provide transportation, and it is common to see a tribal van or shuttle bus pulling up to the Food Distribution stores, letting folks out to get their commodities and waiting while they shop. Indeed, several women I recruited while shopping in the stores had lists from friends or relatives, and they did the shopping for these people as well. As such, picking up commodities rarely looks like picking up a few items today and coming back as often as one likes. Instead, most people pick up their month's worth of foods in one trip. This results in, expectedly, the fresh foods often going bad. For example, Sammy described for me her own negotiating process of getting fresh foods (and letting them go bad), her monthly trip out to McAlester on the tribal van, and why she doesn't ask someone to drive her more regularly.

> Well, sometimes [fresh fruits and vegetables] just do [go bad] because I go ahead and get what I'm allowed and we don't—it's just the two of us—just didn't always get used up every month. If I had a vehicle and I could have

money to make multiple trips over there, that wouldn't happen. . . . The
other thing that the Choctaws provide . . . is they provide transportation
there. . . . [The bus driver], he goes once a month over to McAlester. . . .
I go with him. . . . Mostly the elderly folks—and there are a lot of elderly
Choctaw here, a lot—they just have [the driver] go pick it up for them.
I do the shopping for my aunt who lives here. That's a wonderful thing,
because otherwise I wouldn't have any way to go get my commodities because I couldn't ask somebody. I don't know anybody to ask every month
to take me and supply their gas money and all that kind of thing. (Sammy,
Talihina)

Indeed, the entire shopping experience is a complicated series of ne-
gotiations. Shoppers must negotiate how to divvy up the "poundage"
of their products—fresh vegetables and fruits *or* canned vegetables and
fruits? Frozen meat items *or* canned meat items? When selecting fresh
produce, they open the tied, closed bags of items to trade out foods. For
example, I observed shoppers open bags of two squashes, take out the
smaller squash and trade it for a different, larger squash from another
bag. Because all the bags of squash count as "one pound," they try to get
the most out of that one pound. Moreover, shoppers must negotiate the
day and time they get to the store before the produce is picked over: Fresh
foods are delivered each Wednesday morning, and by Friday morning,
the remaining bags of produce contain the puniest squashes, cabbages,
oranges, etc. Shoppers also must negotiate how to position their items in
their shopping carts *as they shop*, because the *order* of what gets scanned
at check-out matters greatly. For example, shoppers often arranged their
canned vegetables in intentional patterns on the conveyor belt—like one
can of corn, one of green beans, one of peas, then repeated the pattern.
If, say, all the cans of corn were grouped together and scanned first, the
vegetable pound limit for their household might be reached before the
other types of canned vegetables were scanned, leaving the household
with only canned corn for the month. By alternating the order, shoppers
increased their chances of receiving a balanced variety. That leads to the
next negotiation: What to keep or put back when a shopper goes over
their allowed poundage? And what to add when they are under their allowed poundage? I observed this regularly during my fieldwork: A shopper would have either too many pounds of a food item or not enough

pounds of a food item, and the FDPIR staff member, knowing that the shopper would not be back until next month, would offer the shopper the opportunity to run back and grab something. I repeatedly heard staff ask questions like: "Do you wanna grab some hamburger meat? You've got one more meat item left for the month." Or, "You went over on your fruits and vegetables. Do you want to trade anything out?" Or, "You get four UHT boxed milks this month. Do you wanna run 'n' go get them?"

Additionally, the staff checking out shoppers cannot add up the number of a food item and hit Enter. For example, staff cannot scan one can of corn and enter the number "10" for the remaining nine cans of corn. Rather, they must pick up each item and scan it individually to ensure that no mistakes are made. Then, the shopper must reload each item back into the box. In other words, there is a lot of loading, unloading, counting, running back to get food items, and running back to put food items away, such that checking out is not the end of the transaction, but is yet another negotiation of the shopper's food and time—not to mention the time demanded of the other shoppers waiting in line. In sum, FDPIR shoppers must be patient, for there is a lot of waiting and multiple points of negotiation in this food shopping experience. Their time is arguably partial payment for these foods, not only draining hours from their days, but also taking a psychological and cognitive toll (Mani et al. 2013). Where is the dignity and honor in this, when research shows that American poverty and American benefit programs coexist in a "vicious cycle" whereby "unemployment, poverty, health challenges all generate enormous stress and . . . this makes it harder to effectively and efficiently navigate what is needed in order to get help" (Lowrey 2021)?

I spoke with Vanessa, a staff member who works the scanner at one of the FDPIR stores, and who is also a recipient of commodities. As she is both a staff member and client, I asked her about the shopping process. Note the complexity of the shopping interaction and the ways in which she is positioned as "breaking the bad news" to shoppers that they are over their allowed poundage.

> VANESSA: I just kind of—because you don't want to offend anyone and
> make them feel like, that they've done something wrong, like they tried
> to sneak by with a little extra or something. So, I just always make them
> feel like, "Oh, this computer just is so picky." I just feel like, really, the

bad guy that I have to tell them either that "you added wrong" or "you got too many of this." It's kind of like, "Oh, it's no problem—everybody does it. This computer, it just keeps track a little bit better than we add." I just try to make like that.

KASEY: So, I saw this woman wanted grapefruits, but she had a box of raisins, so she had to make the decision what to get, either grapefruit or raisins and—

VANESSA: —switch them out, because you're allowed so many pounds of fruit and so many pounds of vegetables. And probably, the bag of grapefruit would weigh five pounds and raisins count as one [pound]. So, if you have four pounds left at the end of it, and put something else back that weighs one pound, then you can get the five pounds of grapefruit. So, you have to kind of decide what you wanted more at the end of it.

KASEY: I see. Can you walk me thorough how people generally shop?

VANESSA: Usually, they'll get what they want first, and a lot of people will tell me this too, "I'm going to put what I want up here first, and then whatever I have leftover can go towards this, and if I have to put something back"—because they know that it's a weight thing, and it adds up to a certain amount. And then, so whatever is at the end, the leftover, that will be, "I'm okay with putting back." A whole bunch of them know that that's how it goes. So that's what they do. They usually just get everything they really, really want first, and then—they'll have a second pile, and that's the negotiable ones [chuckles].

It seems that the process may get easier for some, however, and the more experienced shoppers are particularly easy to spot. For example, one man strolled into the FDPIR store in Durant when I was there. He said to Vanessa, who was working that day, "Hey Vanessa, what I got left?" and Vanessa replied, "Sixty-one." He nodded, understanding exactly what she meant, but Vanessa elaborated, "Four beans, one bison—but we're out of bison—all your rice, pasta, and soups." But the man was already walking away toward the cardboard boxes, which he selected and put in his shopping cart. The seasoned shoppers stand out, as they communicate in numbers (poundage) instead of items; they move through the four aisles easily and confidently; and they never carry the household shopping list (pound sheet). They stock their carts methodically: cans and juices on the bottom, topped by boxed cheeses, then produce and meats.

Commodity Foods

I am returning for a moment to food memories and women's stories, but more specifically to commodity foods, rations—any foods supplied by the government that are part of their personal or family memories. When asked about food memories, women talked about all sorts of food items, foodways, and food preparations, detailing memories of family gardens (as described earlier, including the growing, picking, canning, and eating of fresh foods); their grandmothers cooking biscuits and gravy for breakfast; older cousins filling up baby bottles with sugar water; and large gatherings of people where food was always shared. One such example was church meetings, where small country churches would rotate hosting other churches once each month, and the hosting church was responsible for cooking huge suppers for the guests. Labor was balanced and divided: The men built a fire outside the church, put a big black pot over the fire, and fried up pig meat while the women worked inside, cooking fried chicken, biscuits, hominy, *banaha*, and all sorts of greens. Women recalled these monthly church suppers with much fondness, especially as beacons of cultural experiences. The suppers were often where (or when) the women recalled "being the most Choctaw," because families and friends gathered and ate together, making it truly "food and fellowship," as one woman described it.

I continued to be moved by these women's thoughtful food memories and humbled that they shared their stories with me, describing in detail the smells, tastes, and textures; the how, where, when, and what people eat; and even inviting me to visit their homes and gardens. I was struck by the fact that their food-related memories always included something related to government food programs (commodities), with many women recalling "Commodities Day," or the day their family received their box of commodity foods. Commodity foods and the everyday practices surrounding them—getting them, cooking with them, and eating them—are deeply woven into these women's lived experiences and memories. These practices aren't just about survival or nutrition; they play a central role in how the women understand and express their Choctaw or Indigenous identity. Whether they were currently receiving commodities or not, they each had memories of and experiences with commodities growing up. Some told stories of their relatives cooking homemade biscuits with

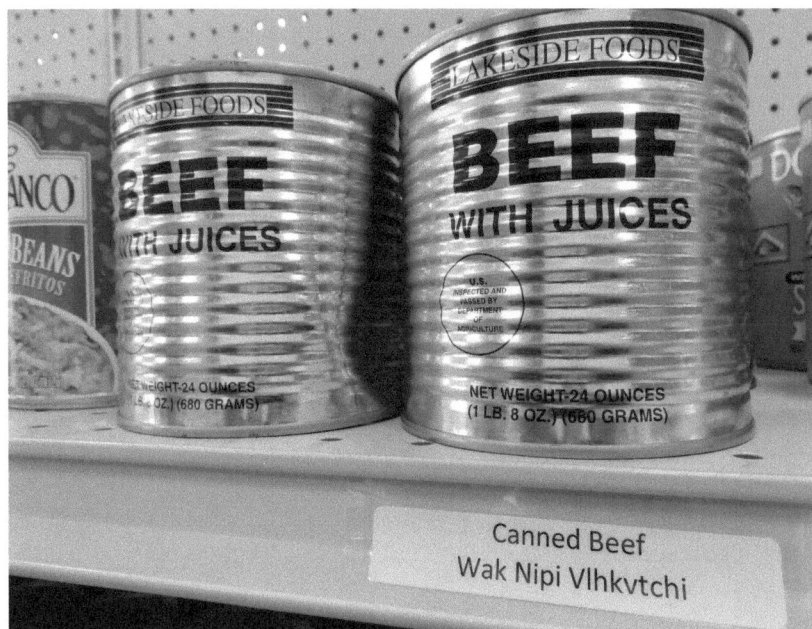

FIGURE 14 Canned beef on a shelf at the FDPIR. Photo by Kasey Jernigan (author).

commodity flour or mixing real eggs with the powdered eggs. Others linked specific foods, such as stewed beef in juices, with being outside in the summertime with their cousins, making picnics with commodities after exploring the woods or swimming in a nearby creek. Commodity-specific foods and the experiences associated with them are intricately woven into the personal and collective memories of these women, shaping their personal identities and informing a shared sense of Indianness. Foods such as flour, cornmeal, pork, and pinto beans are available through the FDPIR program, and women still use many of these staples to prepare cultural Choctaw foods.

As part of the food-related life history interview, I asked what commodities meant to the women in this project. Commodity cheese—the "big block of cheese"—is by far the most popular food item, iconic of commodities, followed by canned meat, dried beans, corn syrup, and pasta, all notable because of quantity; those items "are commodities, and you got lots of it." The commodity foods available are not snacks or

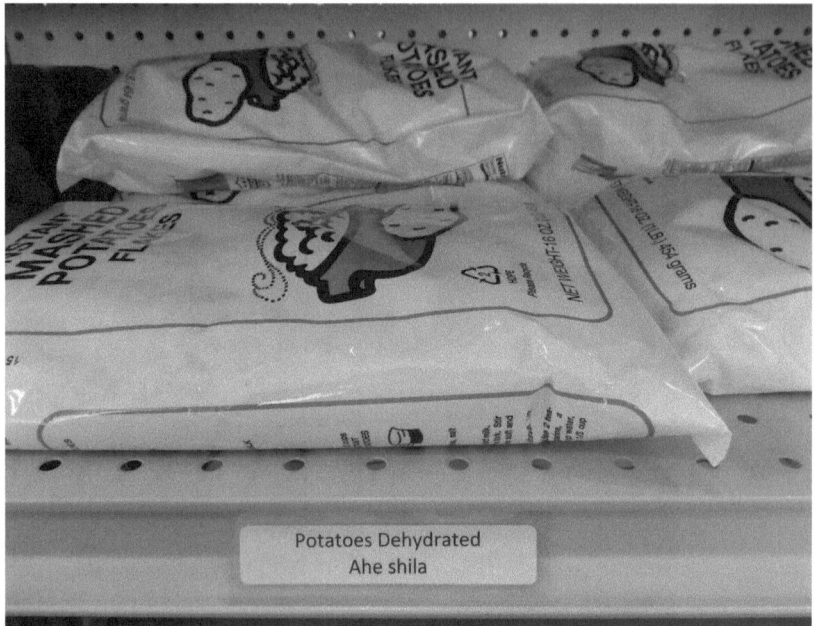

FIGURE 15 Dehydrated potatoes on a shelf. Photo by Kasey Jernigan (author).

quick-grab foods. Rather, they are staples, meant to supplement other foodways, and require cooking and preparation. This is not lost on commodities recipients, many of whom describe needing to get creative with the foods to feed hungry children in between meals. Additionally, for those with children whom they identified as picky eaters, there are rarely alternatives to the foods provided. In other words, while commodities are meant to supplement other foodways, they often serve as a main food source for many families. Since commodities include only specific foods, many women voiced that they would have preferred to get food stamps (i.e., SNAP). They reasoned that with food stamps, they felt they could truly select their own foods. Instead, people who receive commodities often find themselves with foods they do not, cannot, or will not eat.

Women shared that when they sought food assistance through SNAP, they were directed instead to the FDPIR. As stated, the FDPIR does not offer as comprehensive a selection as SNAP. Additionally, many of the available items do not align with diets that doctors recommend for obesity or diabetes. For example, women described taking extra steps to

accommodate their doctor's advice, such as reducing the sodium
content of canned vegetables by
draining and rinsing them, then
reheating with just a touch of
water. One woman described to
me how she would work with the
canned beef.

Well, I would just scrape all the
grease off it, because when you
open that can it's kind of got
grease in it, and I'd just scrape it
all off. And sometimes I wash it
off if I can, and then I just stick it
in the skillet and fry it, let it heat
up, put a little bit of black pepper in it, and sometimes I'll make
sloppy joes out of it, or barbeque
sandwiches.

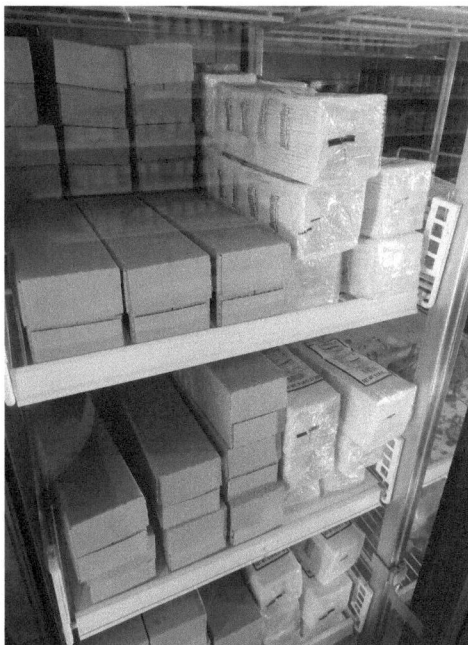

FIGURE 16 Commodity cheese. Photo by Kasey Jernigan (author).

I found it moving when women described the creative ways they managed their commodities. Just as they cared for the fresh foods from their
gardens, many of the women were careful to not waste commodities,
recognizing that although removed from the land through a series of
transactions, these foods still constituted kinship in multiple ways. While
acknowledging that they could potentially sell their surplus commodities
for profit (although this is illegal), some women involved in this project
intentionally opted to share their extras with others in need. They described making care packages with their extra foods for other families,
especially those who were ineligible for FDPIR assistance due to lack of
"proof" of Indigenous affiliation (i.e., a CDIB card) or who lived outside
of the service boundaries of the FDPIR program. As Jessica told me:

I know people that have offered to buy my commodity cheese from me, but
I won't sell it. . . . I had one woman tell me she'd pay me $30 for my entire
block. And I brought her a small chunk, but I told her, "I'm not going it sell

it to you. I'm not giving you any more than that, because that right there will last me over a month . . ." I don't sell or trade any of it, but because we get so much, I'll give it to those in need. I have friends who have three or four children, and they can't afford to feed all of them and pay all of their bills with just her working. So, I'll give her what we—we call them care packages. We make care packages for our friends, and we give them to them. Because we have so much that I don't want it to go to waste. And I know that they aren't able to get any help because they . . . don't have that CDIB card. I do, and I'm more than willing to help someone in need out.

This resonated with me. I grew up in Tulsa, outside of the tribal service areas. My family relied on these care packages from my Choctaw auntie who lived about an hour away from us in the Muscogee Nation and received commodities from their FDPIR. I recall my auntie's visits, the big box of commodities that she and Cousin Raymond always brought with them, and how I would help my mom put the items away in our cabinets. At that time (1980s), the commodity foods were all stamped "USDA" and, with their black and white design, were markedly different from store-bought foods. I remember being embarrassed when my non-Indigenous friends from school would come over, get hungry, and ask for a snack. We'd search the kitchen for something to eat, and they'd always laugh or stare curiously at the absurd commodity foods. How strange and governmental the foods appeared next to the brand-name items like Cheerios! But my family depended on my auntie's care packages, and like the women in this project, these foods also shaped my childhood, informing my nascent understanding of so-called "Indian" foods.

Commodities are generally regarded as not ideal for diabetics, especially the starches such as rice and pastas, but these foods are revered because they channel personal memories of and experiences with commodities while also reflecting the ways that people "eat around here." People have learned to rely heavily on the commodity starches as a method to make meals "stretch" to feed large families and to feed families over longer periods of time. For example, Jessica recalled her grandma's homemade macaroni and cheese, made from commodity pasta and cheese. "Yes, that is the best macaroni and cheese. . . . It's my favorite. It's so not good for you, again, see what I mean? I grew up on nothing good for you. . . . But her mac and cheese was my favorite." Other women talked about these items, mentioning commodity-inspired eating habits they formed in their childhoods, like eating plain macaroni, either boiled or uncooked. These foods—how they were prepared by grandmothers in the past—are still served today and passed on to children, as women describe learning how to cook almost anything with commodities. Take, for example, the bakery mix: It is used to make cakes, pancakes, muffins, bread, or almost anything one can imagine, and its versatility is considered a strength for many families trying to make ends meet. At the same time, its versatility gives women pause about its nutritional value.

The FDPIR has gone to great lengths to improve the nutritional value of commodity foods, as well as making them more inclusive of Indigenous foodways. In addition to more fresh fruits and vegetables, the stores offered blue cornmeal and frozen bison. At the time I was conducting my fieldwork, frozen bison meat was included as a "bonus item," meaning the stores offered it without it counting against a household's monthly allowance for meat. This was part of a larger federal initiative to integrate traditional foods into FDPIR diets (even though bison is not historically a Choctaw food, but rather a staple among tribes in the Great Plains). The women I spoke to had a variety of reactions to the introduction of bison meat as a FDPIR option. Many expressed that the meat has a "wild" flavor, a taste which wasn't entirely to their liking. Despite this, they continued to accept the bison meat and found inventive ways to incorporate it into their meals. Several women I spoke with said they would blend it with ground beef at an equal ratio to make familiar dishes like chili, stews, and burgers more palatable. In a similar creative culinary spirit, women shared that they sometimes combine powdered eggs from commodity packages with actual eggs purchased from grocery stores. This allowed them to recreate the taste and consistency of traditional scrambled eggs while using powdered eggs and conserving real eggs. Others disguised the taste and texture of commodity eggs with lots of ketchup, yet another adaptation that highlights the resourcefulness and ingenuity of Indigenous people when it comes to commodity foods.

The tribe holds monthly cooking workshops at each of the Food Distribution stores, where a dietician spotlights a recipe that incorporates at least one item from the commodity supply, demonstrating how to cook it. "Blue cornmeal tamales" was one recipe featured during my fieldwork, which integrated products such as beef, onions, and cornmeal, all available through the FDPIR program. While blue cornmeal tamales are not originally Choctaw foods, I found it moving yet again to see how women creatively utilize commodities like blue cornmeal to make traditional Choctaw recipes. For instance, cornmeal is a core ingredient in *banaha*, a Choctaw dish similar to tamales. In *banaha*, cornmeal is boiled inside beautifully wrapped corn husks and often served with beans. During conversations I had with one woman, Roberta, she mentioned that she planned to make *banaha* for a friend's birthday and had just picked up her monthly provision of cornmeal. It is not uncommon for people to use their commodities to cook for others—even large meals for the broader community held in tribal spaces. This is another act that embodies the relationality of Choctaw identity—sharing and care-taking are deeply entrenched in Choctaw ways of being, and foods (even commodity foods that come from violent neoliberal policies disguised as "care" that work to make invisible the government's role in Indigenous food inequities and health disparities) are an important part of the kinship, connection, and relationality that bring people together. I include Roberta's words here, as I do not want to paraphrase their beautiful simplicity.

> I love to cook, and so I just learned how to make the traditional Choctaw *banaha*, which is the cornmeal rolled in the corn shucks. . . . That's why I got a bunch of cornmeal today, is because I got a huge order for next week for the Choctaw senior citizens. So, I'm going to be making a bunch of *banaha* next Wednesday. . . . I'm going to make it and go to the center with it because they were asking if I could make it for one of our elders, who is ninety-four. I believe she's in that calendar there [the tribe's monthly calendar featuring tribal citizens]. It'll be her birthday, and so I am making it for her.

Eating is a deeply social act intimately associated with identity, with decades of research confirming the profound relationships between food and individual and group identities (Beardsworth and Keil 1997; Counihan and Van Esterik 2012; Garine 1995; Meigs 1997; Roy 2006). Throughout the women's stories, food was used in all social relations and, as Pilcher (2012) notes, "food habits" are components of tiny crossroads of history. Food choices at once express and show a sense of belonging (to a people, a nation) and of distinguishment (from Others)—all from a personal, social, and political perspective (Roy 2006; Counihan 1999). Furthermore, food habits and cuisines are seen as constructs, only fully comprehensible through the lens of both their current and historical socio-economic and political contexts. It is clear that FDPIR recipients' food habits extend beyond mere individual choice and are instead intricately co-created through the political act(s) of acquiring, cooking, sharing, depending on, eating, and even enjoying commodities (Roy 2006). Commodities (and the many political acts associated with them) create and build social alliances, contributing to the development of social solidarity, which serves to define "who is who" (Roy 2006).

The women in this research insisted that commodities are not traditional Choctaw foods (they are not culturally Choctaw, and our ancestors would not know what a lot of these food stuffs were); however, commodities (and the related political acts of acquiring them and so on) are described, in part, as what it means to be Choctaw. That is, for these women, being Choctaw involves grappling in one way or another with the effects and affects of settler colonialism. They identified poverty, racism, chronic health diseases (specifically diabetes and obesity), dependence on commodity foods, and an abundance of processed and unhealthy foods. One woman described these interconnected experiences as:

Something of a kinship that you don't have with the "paper Indians."[4] [Commodities are] not a cultural thing, because we didn't—culturally, we didn't have that food. We didn't subsist on the food items that are—the food that we grew up eating. You had to go out and get your food. You had to grow your food. . . . And somewhere along the way we forgot how to feed ourselves from the earth. And we got the commodities, and we learned all about them loaves of bread and starchy food. And, it was cheap, I guess. That's how we all—I can speak for a traditional Choctaw way. There's a big difference between traditional Choctaws and Choctaws that aren't Choctaws, you know what I mean? They probably grew up eating differently but obesity, diabetes, they are very much a part of our life now [for traditional Choctaws]. Yes, absolutely.

Women shared inside jokes about commodity foods, highlighting how familiarity with, and reliance upon, particular commodity foods serves as signifiers of authenticity, distinguishing those who really grew up "Indian" from those who, presumably, did not, and revealing the ways in which commodities work to allow individuals to acknowledge themselves as members of the same group. Jessica casually laughed with me about commodities, playfully stating, "I mean we make jokes about commodity stuff. If you don't know what canned beef is, then you didn't grow up Indian." Others claimed commodity cheese is real "Indian food" because it's only available through the FDPIR, but also because settler colonial assimilation policies worked so well to eliminate Choctaw foodways and knowledge of these foodways and foods—at the very least, knowledge of how to prepare foods. Jessica echoed a sentiment that many others shared with me too: "Commodities is my Indian food, I guess."

Undoubtedly, commodities have become intertwined with the stereotype of poverty, often perceived as shorthand for the "poor Indian" image or the notion of Indigenous people being overly dependent and given everything for free. They find themselves continually educating others that these "benefits" were originally agreed upon in treaties as part of land exchanges for healthcare and education. Yet commodities as symbols of poverty, and particularly Indian poverty, carry significant implications and make up much of the local discourse around obesity and indigeneity. Women described common outside perspectives of Indians as poor, dependent, lazy, fat, drunk, unemployed, given everything from the government, and so on. Sammy shared with me:

> Outsiders think of it that way. Just another drunk, and just another fat, lazy Indian . . . because they don't work. They don't work because they're given everything or [laughs] not given everything, given so little. Like I said, they gave us 160 acres per person of land that already belonged to us, for heaven sakes! And then turned around and took it away from us.

Another woman, Vivian, agreed. "Commodities, it's not only Native Americans, it's also based on income. You have to be below a certain amount of income in order to get commodities. So, I think that right there kind of labels—and I hate labeling people, but that labels you as someone who is poor and unable to feed your family."

These perspectives continue to harm and threaten Choctaws in a variety of ways, and they also are pivotal components of violent neoliberal colonial bureaucracy, which encompasses not just instances of direct physical violence (e.g., genocidal boarding schools and removal of children from their families), but also the perpetuation of structural inequalities. This includes insufficient access to essential services and provisions such as nutritious food, healthcare, safe housing, and wellness facilities. Additionally, they involve symbolic and insidious forms of harm, such as the regulation and stigmatization of personal identity or creating environments conducive to the internalization of violence.

Obesity: Choctaw Women's Perspectives

Although obesity is a growing concern worldwide, with an expanding body of research dedicated to understanding its multiple dimensions, there remains a significant gap in the literature concerning the specific experiences and perceptions of obesity among Indigenous populations. This is concerning for multiple reasons, including the stark disparity in obesity rates (and related conditions) between Indigenous and non-Indigenous populations, which suggests that existing public health strategies (predominantly developed from non-Indigenous perspectives) have been largely ineffectual. The multifaceted nature of obesity is well-documented, encompassing physiological, behavioral, psychological, and environmental factors. Yet, prevailing public health messages for weight management predominantly emphasize personal responsibility narratives centered on dieting, caloric restriction, and exercise. While these approaches are well-intentioned, they often evoke feelings of guilt and failure when the desired outcomes are not achieved. More, such messages fail to consider the sociocultural contexts of Indigenous communities, underscoring the need for further research that incorporates these dimensions. In this section, I offer Choctaw understandings of obesity from the research project to bridge the existing research gap by exploring intrinsic factors specific to Choctaw interpretations of obesity. This nuanced understanding is vital for developing more effective intervention strategies that resonate with both individual and collective experiences of obesity and well-being among Choctaws and Indigenous peoples more generally.

Choctaw Understandings of Obesity: Indians Like to Eat

As part of this project, I asked participants to share how they perceived their current body size using the Body Image Assessment instrument (Williamson et al. 2000).[5] To administer the scale, the cards (each with a figure of a different size) were shuffled and presented in random order. Women were instructed to select the silhouette that most accurately depicted their body size as they perceived it to be. This was an interesting activity, as it opened dialogue around ideal body sizes, notions of "healthy" and "unhealthy" body sizes, Choctaw bodies, and white bodies.[6]

For these women, the term *obesity* means "really, really fat," "overly fat," or "waddle, waddle fat," but it was difficult to pin down a specific size meant by these descriptors. Obesity, although widely prevalent, seemed to be difficult for them to definitively label. They were surrounded by fat people, as they commented repeatedly, and even described themselves as "overweight," or "a little bit heavy," yet few people could objectively state what was obese and what was not. Indeed, many of them were surprised to learn that they are, themselves, considered obese or morbidly obese by medical standards. Findings from the Body Image Assessment Scale (BIA-O),[7] which was designed for use with persons ranging from very thin to very obese, correspond with the qualitative data. That is, participants overall perceived their current body sizes at a mean score of 9.6 (± 3.4), which is just between the "normal" and "overweight" body size ranges. Yet, almost two-thirds of the sample (63 percent, n = 31) was considered "obese" based on their body mass index (BMI).[8] In fact, only five participants perceived their current body size as "obese," and approximately half (n = 20) perceived their body size as "normal" (while only four participants fell into the "normal" weight category based on their BMIs).

Women overwhelmingly scored what they perceive to be healthy and unhealthy body sizes within the appropriate ranges.[9] The majority of women indicated that the body sizes on both extremes of the scale (i.e., very thin and very obese) were equally unhealthy, and many selected both or more to indicate unhealthy body sizes. They overwhelmingly perceived Choctaw women to have larger bodies than non-Choctaws (i.e., white women). The perceived mean size of Choctaw women's bodies was 10.8 (± 2.3), or in the "overweight" category, while the perceived mean size of white women's bodies was 7.14 (± 2.5), or in the "normal" category. These data suggest that Choctaws do perceive themselves to be generally larger than their white counterparts. However, they also perceive their current body sizes to be smaller than they actually are. This was an incredibly rich exercise, because conversations pointed to the complexity and multiple valences of obesity. For example, women distinguished between urban white and rural white women, indicating that the former are generally thinner and more "in shape," whereas the latter "look like us." Thus, they correlated obesity with where one lives and one's socioeconomic status. Interestingly, however, no one made this distinction among urban and rural Choctaw women.

In addition to the terms "obese" and "overweight," women used several local terms for fat bodies, including "thick," "big-boned," "large," and "healthy." The term "healthy" has long been a colloquial euphemism for "fat" within Choctaw communities. Carmen shared that she considers herself "healthy" now because that's the term used for being overweight, noting that "healthy" is essentially a more polite way of saying fat. She likes to say about herself, "I'm *very* healthy," as a way to acknowledge that she is obese and sensitive to the multiple meanings of fatness and healthiness. Talking about her size, she states, "Even my husband agrees, saying, 'Yes, you're healthy, and so am I.'" She clarifies that her husband is in fact not overweight, but rather, "He has a little belly, but in reality, that's healthy and I'm plus-sized." That is, for Choctaws and within Choctaw understandings of what is a healthy body, a little belly is fine, normal, and healthy. To summarize, the term "fat" sometimes carries pejorative connotations, leading individuals to prefer softer, more acceptable phrases when in certain company. These terms also differentiate a particular notion of being overweight where health issues are absent, often described as "carrying their weight well" (e.g., "a little belly"), indicating ongoing activity and apparent healthiness. Among other Choctaws, however, the term "fat" is used affectionately, and comments on weight and body size are often made in a good-natured teasing context, serving as a form of lighthearted banter with familiar insiders of the community. For example, elder women are affectionately called "short, fat, and jolly," pointing to a cultural norm of endearment and humor when coming from other Indians; this would be perceived differently if expressed by non-Natives.

This dynamic highlights the nuanced understanding of such interactions within the community, where in-group familiarity and mutual comprehension shape the acceptability of these remarks.

Among *Chahta anumpa* speakers, there was lots of laughter about how they use *Chahta* words for "big" (*chito*), "fat" (*nia*), and "lard" or "grease" (*bila*) to describe fat bodies, especially in a playful way. Roberta was delighted to share this quip with me:

> *Chito*, which means "big" in Choctaw. "Oh, they're *chito*," or we'll say, "*Chiiiiii-tooooo*," where the longer you sound it out, the more it means, you know, the fatter they are. . . . When someone comes by, we'll go "*chito*," [whispers], like that. And everyone will start giggling, "Yeah, that's a big boy [chuckles]." We hear that a lot, and because we say it in Choctaw, you'd just kind of say it in a teasing way, under voice, with your mouth hidden like that [covers mouth, laughs].

Women describe a prevalent "*Indian* body type" among Choctaws (men and women both), characterized by a larger midsection, wide hips, and "skinny little arms and legs." This notion extends to the observation that weight among Choctaw women is predominantly carried in the torso rather than the hips and thighs, a curvy physicality that they typically associate with white women and sometimes envied in their youth. Sammy shared an experience of everyday violence related to her body shape: A colleague in Tulsa derogatorily called her a "blanket ass." This is an expression stemming from a couple of racist tropes about Native women: how Indian women used to wrap themselves in blankets and the stereotype that Indian women do not have curvy butts but instead have flat, wide butts (like an Indian blanket).

Despite widespread and generalized ideas about Choctaw women's bodies as "short and squatty," these women largely acknowledged that they never viewed themselves as overweight simply because of their body types; however, some did express a longing for curvy, hourglass figures they associated with non-Indigenous women. Vivian noted a shift in perceptions of Native women's bodies, particularly among the Choctaws, indicating that current stereotypes favor a fuller figure over traditional portrayals of slender Native women: "When you think of Native Americans, especially Choctaw, you think of a more rounded figure. You don't

TABLE 3 Summary of participants' self-reported health information

Criteria	Sample Population N = 49
Health in general	
Excellent	0
Very good	6 (12%)
Good	24 (49%)
Fair	13 (27%)
Poor	3 (6%)
No answer	3 (6%)
Height mean ± SD (in inches) [Range]	64.3 ± 3.3 [53–72]
Weight mean ± SD (in pounds) [Range]	200.3 ± 47.6 [122.7–308.2]
Waist Circumference mean ± SD (in inches) [Range]	44.6 ±7 [31–57.5]
BMI [Range]	[18.3–52]
Underweight (< 18.5)	1 (2%)
Normal (18.5–24.9)	4 (8%)
Overweight (25–29.9)	11 (22%)
Obese (30 +)	31 (63%)
Obese I (30–34.9)	11 (22%)
Obese II (35–39.9)	9 (18%)
Obese III (40 +)	11 (22%)

Note: Percentages (%) are rounded.

think of the stereotypical long black hair, skinny Indian girl. You think of the more rotund Indian girl."

Among the women interviewed, what they considered an ideal body size hovered around a size twelve or fourteen, perceived as both healthy and an attainable goal, while the desire for thinness was notably absent. Many women associated weight loss with challenging life experiences, observing that stress and adversity could significantly impact their appetites. A leaner body was often linked to illness or economic hardship, indicating that concerns over thinner bodies were not solely aesthetic but rather intertwined with health and socio-economic status. For example, one woman shared her personal experience of weight loss following the bereavement of her grandson, during which she stopped eating and experienced significant weight loss before being prescribed antidepressants, which worked to restore her appetite. Another woman echoed similar sentiments, expressing a preference for "thickness" rather than embracing thinness, which she equated with unhealthiness and frailty.

She reminisced about wearing a pair of jeans sized fourteen, considering it a comfortable and healthy weight—a perspective that underscored the women's broader views on body image and wellness.

Interestingly, women noted a shift in the rationale for thinness, highlighting what they understood as "right" and "wrong" reasons to lose weight. They described how weight loss and thin bodies are now viewed as a reflection of health and self-care, rather than simply a beauty standard. This perspective was bolstered by participants' comments associating attainable thinness with stress or illness. Nelly Coyote, the woman introduced in chapter 3, articulated this transition by describing how, in the past, she wanted to be thin so she would be considered beautiful. But now, the emphasis seemed to be on health, and it felt like a significant change, focusing on wellness. Women commented on the societal perceptions linked to thinness for "appropriate" reasons, indicating that when they were perceived as thin *and* healthy—registered as lifestyle changes such as weight loss through focused diet, exercise, and self-care practices—the ways they were treated changed. Fat bodies faced assumptions of neglect concerning self-care, while thinner bodies received acknowledgment for apparent health consciousness. Carmen's experience of substantial weight loss through focused diet, exercise, and self-care practices reflects the repercussions of this change. She was perceived as "active" and "athletic," leading to positive social interactions and perceptions of youthfulness. This positivity catalyzed further self-improvements, such as investing in personal grooming and attire, affirming her progression to a social image embodying the "right" reasons for thinness—health and self-care, ultimately receiving different forms of acceptance and admiration.

Indeed, all the women who were part of this research articulated a nuanced understanding of the determinants of obesity, their insights aligning with widely recognized factors. They referenced lack of physical activity, unhealthy dietary habits, a preference for fried foods, and eating. This last aspect, characterized as a "Native appetite," is notably prominent at social gatherings such as Indian church dinners. Food is central at these events, and everyone is encouraged to eat well (i.e., eat a lot). Tables brim with huge servings of an array of dishes, and people return to the table for seconds and thirds, filling their plates with fry bread, Indian tacos, chicken-fried steak, fried potatoes, and pasta salads, while "the salad somebody brought would be the last to go, or still around once everybody's done eating." It's not uncommon for a diabetic to "just take extra insulin if he eats bad." The women described a type of dietary restraint among the non-Natives at these events, contrasting it with local Choctaw norms. For example, one woman described her white pastor's disciplined eating, noting his much smaller portion sizes compared to the Choctaws and his preference for the salad (which is what his wife usually brought to share). Carmen recounted a local legend about the healthcare implications following these communal feasts.

> I always heard that at camp [church] meetings and things like that—a lot of Indian churches they have Indian foods, and they could always tell when there was a camp meeting because the clinics would be full that Monday [laughter]. Because a lot of Indians would go to the camp meetings and just eat all this Indian food and make themselves sick or their blood pressure go up and everything.

Economic factors were also recognized as relevant, with women connecting poverty to obesity: Financial constraints limit access to nutritious foods, leaving families reliant on affordable, processed options like "bologna and bread and processed cheese." They identified this double bind as jeopardizing their health because of what they could afford. In other words, they found themselves in the impossible situation of having to choose between eating unhealthily or not eating at all. Linked in their narratives about poverty was stress, particularly the stress associated with caregiving responsibilities and domestic challenges. Women often shoulder the responsibility of maintaining family cohesion and providing care for grandchildren while their children are either working, living elsewhere, or otherwise unable to parent due to a variety of circumstances. Caregiving is now clearly recognized as a significant source of stress across age, gender, ethnicity, and types of illnesses. This stress emerges from both primary and secondary stressors and includes pressure from supporting roles and responsibilities beyond the caregiving itself, leading to a reduced sense of control over one's own life. Additionally, some women attributed obesity to genetic factors, citing family histories characterized by large body types. Despite having made efforts to lose weight, many women reported being unsuccessful and explored the underlying reasons for their inability to achieve weight loss. Furthermore, they recognized the interplay between obesity and other health conditions, such as thyroid disorders, polycystic ovarian syndrome, diabetes, and unexplained hereditary ailments. This nexus of health issues raised concerns primarily about the well-being of their children and grandchildren. Such perspectives were often intertwined with a fatalistic outlook on obesity and diabetes, manifesting in the belief that these conditions are inevitable among Indians and leading to a sense of resignation that "diabetes is in our genes."

Discussions with the women articulated a direct correlation between historical trauma—such as the loss of land and forced displacement—and the structural violence that manifests as reliance on commodity foods. They explicitly linked commodity foods as a contributing factor to the prevalence of obesity within their communities today. But they discussed how historical events associated with forced removal (i.e., rations during and after relocation, disruption of localized knowledge around food sources, loss of families, loss of community, all the death that transpired, etc.) induced significant cultural upheaval, often described in the literature as "culture shock" or "cosmological grief" (Scheder 2006:45). Their narratives also highlighted experiences of alcoholism, physical violence, shame, and racism, intricately linked to the history of boarding schools, language loss, disrupted parenting traditions, relocation, and lost ways of knowing and being. Women linked the introduction of processed foods and sugars, thought to have been foreign to Indigenous peoples pre-contact, with a drastic health transformation that they now saw as rampant obesity, diabetes, and hypertension. They described the separation from ancestral lands and loss of traditional farming practices as important contributors to current Choctaw health crises, suggesting cultural disorientation due to removal and relocation. Their explanatory models for obesity were vast yet specific and included the introduction of western diets such as alcohol and sugar; disrupted traditional eating patterns which foster dependence on unhealthy foods often associated with poverty; and drastic dietary shifts accompanying relocation that may have overwhelmed their bodies' adaptive capacities, possibly contributing to diabetes and other diet-related health issues.

Indeed, these women, like Choctaws in general, were well aware of the significance of a healthy diet and exercise in maintaining a normal weight, but this form of biocitizenship (Greenhalgh and Carney 2014) that controls and disciplines bodies by framing obesity as a moral and individual failure led them to believe they deserved their circumstances. Indeed, this blaming of Indigenous peoples for the obesity epidemic in Indian communities aligns with the logics of settler-colonialism that seek to eliminate Natives and represents yet another form of symbolic violence that contributes to the "slow death" (Berlant 2007) of Natives, all while exacerbating their health risks by neglecting the underlying causes of obesity and related conditions.

The lived experiences of obese Choctaw women often entail predictable discomfort and societal challenges, including being mistaken as pregnant or facing difficulties in clothing shopping and being unable to find well-fitting clothes. The women also described everyday challenges like fitting into desks, using seatbelts, navigating narrow shopping aisles, and even securing employment. They were aware of public perceptions that associate fat bodies with poor health and self-care, perpetuating stigmatizing stereotypes. On the other hand, fat bodies are intertwined with notions of solidarity and acceptance within their own families and communities, particularly through communal eating practices. Sharing meals and eating together was described as intrinsic to Choctaw ways of being, and the types and quantities of food consumed were agreed to contribute to obesity's being so common. Some women even joked about enabling each other to overeat and overeat unhealthy foods. For example, Sherry described her experiences at Indian church, describing the gatherings that involve ample servings of food.

> They have all this food out there, and they give you a plate. What is it? An eight-inch plate, maybe. By the time that you get through that line, your plate is a tower. It's about eight inches high. Yes, you are just pushing the food down so it won't fall off. Indians like to eat. They like the fellowship and our churches; I was telling the pastor, the other day I said, "The only way I'm going to lose weight is to quit coming to church" [laughter]. He said, "You can't do that." But, every time you turn around, they're eating.

This sentiment was echoed by others who observed that the prevalence of obesity is partly due to eating habits established in childhood and noting that fried foods are synonymous with Choctaw culture, making dietary change challenging. There is a normalization of obesity—"people don't even think anything about it [obesity]"—and in such small communities, some "have been three hundred pounds" for as long as others have known them, leading to an acceptance of larger body sizes. Lastly, women described how their social circles would minimize concerns over their weight gain, suggesting a communal approach to body perception.

The act of eating itself demands detailed exploration, as conversations with women reveal its multifunctional role as an act of hospitality, cultivating community, creating shared memories, and marking being together. Eating together is often the time when stories are told, when youth learn about their family histories and their places in the world. Carmen described how her son and his grandfather connect while sharing food; her son, despite his young age, absorbs his grandfather's stories, some heavy and complicated, covering themes of racism, violence, and segregation. The imparting of these stories during mealtime suggests that the sharing of food and conversations functions as a dynamic way of teaching and relating, promoting intergenerational cultural continuity. Feeding others is also a vital theme in the context of eating. Women recounted multiple instances of engaging in mutual care through food: Women cook together, deliver meals and foods to those in need, and share whatever food resources they have. Women told stories of how, in their childhoods, being Choctaw meant taking part in a close-knit community, typically centered around Indian church, and having visitors pop in unscheduled, where sharing whatever foods you had was customary. This is often described as "the Choctaw way."

The centrality of food at gatherings was echoed across women, with enjoyment coming from the food as much as the presence and participation of lots of people, creating a joyful, fun, communal atmosphere.[10] The act of eating transcends just consumption; it is intertwined with social interaction. However, it is clear that this culturally significant practice of eating together is also intricately linked to the prevalence of obesity, as the emphasis on "sharing," "eating," "fellowshipping," and "getting full" remains important, with the refrain that "Indians like to eat" resonating among participants.

Conclusion

In general, the women I spoke with challenged the notion that being fat can be simply called an "Indian thing." However, there was a consensus that Choctaws, and Indians in general, often struggle with issues of (and related to) obesity. They argued that this is not merely a cultural characteristic but rather a manifestation of broader socio-economic hardships, including struggle, poverty, and discrimination, which have become markers of Choctaw experiences, both lived and inherited, and Indianness more broadly. They noted that, while being fat is not necessarily a an "Indian thing," Indians are "pretty fat." Factors contributing to this include dietary preferences for fried and unhealthy foods, diminished engagement in gardening and farming, and reduced physical activity. Furthermore, the discussions revealed that Choctaw women recognize the larger historical, social, and political-economic influences on contemporary obesity rates. One noted factor is the loss of land, which curtails opportunities for gardening and food self-sufficiency. Additionally, the historical and continued need for the food distribution program has perpetuated stereotypes of dependency and laziness, while pervasive health disparities, such as diabetes, have worked to create a fatalistic mindset toward such illnesses. Despite the prevalence of obesity, participants acknowledged that "food and fellowship" remain central to Choctaw identity, with gatherings heavily emphasizing the importance of abundance and fulfillment. Importantly, being fat is not necessarily perceived as negative, nor is the presence of obesity-related diabetes necessarily viewed as detrimental—obesity and diabetes are perceived as inevitable. However, Choctaws do recognize the adverse outcomes of unmanaged diabetes, such as blindness and amputation, as negative.

Commodity foods significantly constitute both the everyday and traditional diets for Choctaws, and they are deeply woven into the women's individual and collective food-related memories. The women agreed that commodities—receiving them, depending on them, sharing them, and cooking with them, either in the past or present—make up part of what it means to be Indian today. However, they noted that struggle, poverty, and discrimination are also part of Indian identity, and these experiences go hand-in-hand. In other words, to receive, depend on, share, and cook with commodities symbolizes the complex experiences of struggle, poverty, and discrimination that are products of "being Indian in a white world."

Roy (2006) argues that the analysis of changes in food habits and its contemporary and daily expression reveals the creative power of those who, on a daily basis, build viable universes and moments of happiness with contemporary materials such as commodities. These women, and Choctaws in general, indeed experience "moments of joy" in their daily lives and a locally conceptualized and operationalized condition of health and wellbeing through their actions and relationships. In his work with the Canadian Innu, Roy (2006:182) argues that the "act of eating" is a social and political act of recognition and differentiation, illustrating how the Innu associate healthy foods with "white foods," prompting the notion of an Innu "killer identity" that is closely linked to historical and current conditions of exclusion from mainstream society. Similarly, Saethre (2013) illustrates how diabetes is used as an idiom, identity, and tool of contestation through which Indigenous Australians argue for recognition and rights in an environment of pervasive racial disparity. In this research, Choctaws identified obesity and the sequelae of chronic health problems as major concerns, not necessarily for reasons the public health establishment would assume, but rather for the historical, social, and political-economic dimensions responsible for the origin of these health conditions. Changes in foods and foodways and their relationship to the body are all involved in the geneses of obesity among Choctaws and are closely associated with the process of Indigenous relationality and identity creation. This identity is, on the one hand, the result of legitimate resistance and, on the other hand, a response to demands for distinct indigeneity, a distinct Indigenous identity (Povinelli 2002), but it is always traced as health inequities rooted in longstanding relationships between Indigenous people, non-Indigenous settlers, and illness (Jones 2004).

Conclusion

An embodied heritage framework offers an approach, informed by Native American Indigenous studies and critical biocultural anthropology, for understanding the ways in which obesity among Oklahoma Choctaws intersects with historical trauma; structural, symbolic, and everyday violence; and social processes of heritage and identity. These key components provide a general framework to critically interpret the biocultural interactions behind the disproportionate distribution and escalation of obesity among Choctaws in the past four decades. Yet this orientation extends well beyond the experiences of Choctaws in southeastern Oklahoma and elucidates the critical point of meaning-making that functions around obesity and its intersections with both the past and present among Native Americans more generally.

The introduction positions embodied heritage as a departure from biomedical paradigms that frame obesity as an individual condition, instead emphasizing the entanglement of historical trauma; structural, symbolic, and everyday violence; and ongoing social processes of identity and heritage. From the outset, the book argues that Choctaw women's experiences of obesity are inseparable from larger systems of political economy, settler colonialism, and forced dependence on government commodities, all of which shape the material realities of their food choices and health outcomes. The framework extends beyond the Choctaw Nation, offering insights into how Native American communities broadly navigate and reinterpret historical trauma in relation to health.

Throughout previous chapters, I describe how Choctaw women make sense of their experiences of obesity and related conditions in southeastern Oklahoma. I describe how such experiences are interlinked with the ways in which historical trauma is used as a public narrative (Mohatt et al. 2014) to make sense of obesity and how that interacts with macro-level forces of history, political economy, and contemporary forms of violence, as well as heritage narratives evoked to underpin individual and group identity. The chapters recount food-centered life stories of women who personify the complexity of these intersections, revealing the interconnections of historical trauma; structural, symbolic, and everyday violence; heritage; identity; and obesity. These women's stories offer a narrative view of individualized behaviors, experiences, meaning-making, and heritage-making associated with food, obesity, and identity. As such, these lived experiences cannot be dissociated from the historical, political-economic, and social inequalities that shape them, or the impact that such experiences have on escalating rates of obesity (and diabetes).

Along the way, I examine the key components of obesity within the embodied heritage framework, including historical trauma; structural, symbolic, and everyday violence; heritage; and identity and illustrate how each entity is inextricably linked with the others. I argue that it is difficult to separate the "self" from larger historical, political-economic, and social contexts, as these macro-forces facilitate individual ways of being in the world. I suggest that indigeneity connected with obesity is an important manifestation of historical, political-economic, and social realities that cannot be understood apart from social demands for (Indian) authenticity. Even more, individual experiences must be realized as part of a larger social and political system in which Indigenous peoples are largely held to a level of distinction and cultural continuity not demanded of others (Barker 2011; Cattelino 2010; Dennison 2012; Povinelli 2002), contributing to creative engagements with these demands for authenticity. One such approach is the obesity-identity interface that links foods, foodways, and health within a framework that considers the historical, political-economical, and socio-cultural forces that shaped them. Embodied heritage focuses on meaning-making, personal and public narratives, and cultural identities. Put simply, an embodied heritage framework argues that health is contingent on one's social, economic, historical, cultural, and political position *and* the structures of meaning that make sense of this personal and embodied experience.

Throughout this work, narrative emerges as both the means and the method through which Choctaw women articulate their lived experiences, revealing a grounded theory of historical trauma and contemporary violence in relation to foodways, heritage, culture, and identity. Storytelling is not merely a reflection on the past but an active engagement with the present, a way of making sense of ongoing and felt disparities in health and food security, and a means of shaping the future through Choctaw cultural survivance. The embodied heritage framework introduced in this book serves as a theoretical and methodological lens for understanding how narratives unfold—how history is not just recalled but experienced and embodied in the everyday realities of Choctaw women and how these are related to health.

I hope the findings from this project work to demonstrate that *how* people think about their personal and collective pasts directly affects their health outcomes. Adding to other studies that underscore the value of understanding how (and which) representations of the past are evoked and used to explain health (Blackstock et al. 2006; Ferreira and Lang 2006; Mohatt et al. 2014; Scheder 2006; Whitbeck et al. 2004), the findings from this project come together to illustrate that Choctaws recall past traumatic events both as public narrative and personal experiences as a way to make sense of what they identify in the present: interrupted traditions and reimagined Choctaw culture expressed in the day-to-day. This finding is essential because it informs local narratives that explain health inequities, specifically obesity and related conditions. Rather than simply stating that obesity is "a marker of Indianness," Choctaw women understand their health not as markers of personal failure but as embodiment of struggle, poverty, and discrimination; experiences that are marked by poor food environments and a continued dependence on government-supplied foods, as well as cultural and material dispossession (i.e., loss of land, language, traditions, cultural expressions, knowledge and stories, and more). Their reflections challenge dominant public health discourses that pathologize Indigenous bodies, instead offering a framework where health disparities are understood as material consequences of historical trauma, contemporary forms of violence, and the linked processes of identity- and heritage-making.

Implications for Embodied Heritage

In the Choctaw Nation and across Indian Country, there were (and continue to be) substantially greater rates of COVID-19 mortality among Indians, with deaths credited to the high prevalence of obesity. Such discourses obscure deep-seated historical and ongoing injustices that shape these data, these present realities. Narratives of risk often neglect to address how the legacies of settler colonialism and structural violence have entrenched the very disparities that persist today, contributing to disproportionate rates of COVID-related fatalities among Indigenous peoples. Instead of just attributing vulnerability to individual health conditions like obesity, it is important to understand how historical processes and systemic inequities have cultivated environments where Indigenous peoples face higher susceptibility to pandemics.

The interviews for this project were conducted before the onset of the COVID-19 pandemic in early 2020, which altered the way of life for billions of people across the globe. COVID-19 continues to have a discursive grip on some bodies more than others. Here is the statistical nightmare: The latest research shows that for the first time in more than a century, life expectancy (the most basic measure of the health of a population) of all Americans dropped due to the pandemic. For Native Americans, it dropped by as much as six and a half years, more than double the numbers in white America and equivalent to life expectancy figures for all Americans in 1944.[1] In 2020 alone, life expectancy for Natives dropped by four years and is now lower than that of every country in the Americas except Haiti (Andrasfay and Goldman 2021; Rabin 2022). During the height of the pandemic, Indigenous peoples in the United States were the most disproportionately impacted by COVID-19, nearly three times as likely to be hospitalized with the disease and more than twice as likely to die of it. The case rate has been 50 percent higher among Natives than among white Americans, and it is safe to say that these figures are likely lower than the reality, because death certificates often misclassify Native peoples (settler-colonialism's final sleight-of-hand, whereby one is born Native but dies white).

These data don't even attempt to account for the felt experiences of suffering, with families losing members in the double digits: aunties, uncles, grandmothers, grandfathers, sisters, brothers, mothers, fathers, children, and so on (you get the picture). These aren't just family members we've lost; they're knowledge holders, dressmakers, artists, *Chahta anumpa* speakers, elders, and other important people in our communities. Each death is a loss of knowledge, loss of language, loss of ways, connections, relations, parts of who we are and how we know who we are— gone. Burial grounds full, funerals occurring multiple times a day, family members saying goodbye from inside their cars or over Zoom, funeral rites left undone, spirits prevented from journeying home. A pandemic is a biosocial event that facilitates dispossession, a biosocial process of becoming dispossessed (Belcourt 2018). Scholars, epidemiologists, and federal researchers were slow to understand the extent of the disaster, and they simply claimed "pre-existing conditions" as explanation, specifically the extraordinarily high rates of obesity and diabetes, but also alcoholism, liver damage, overdoses, homicide, respiratory illnesses, and so on—"pre-existing conditions" that are notoriously prevalent in Indian communities. Some researchers further linked these "pre-existing conditions" with poverty, contaminated and/or lack of running water, and the tragically underfunded Indian Health Services. But, as Belcourt (2018) reminds us, when a people are hailed as sick over and over again, considered predisposed to these conditions of dispossession, it is indigeneity that materializes as pathogenic in regard to histories of settler colonialism, and fat bodies are always an easy target. Rendered "willfully deviant" as Margery Fee (2006) argues, "as if they were deserving of whatever misfortune befalls them," fat bodies as a risk factor for COVID is also a way of chalking up COVID-related morbidity and mortality as a biological tragedy waiting to happen: the source of the problem firmly situated in Indigenous peoples themselves, a run-of-the mill form of Indigenous self-destruction, rather than a corporeal haunting of empire, civilization, and progress (Belcourt 2018).

As described in the introduction, I began this research with personal interest in unraveling the relationships between health outcomes and historical trauma. My family's experiences with dispossession, Indian boarding schools, violence, and the profound impacts of assimilation policies that have reverberated across generations inspired my anthropological examination of historical trauma. In collaboration with Choctaw tribal citizens across Oklahoma, we focused on obesity and related conditions. Commonly expressed was concern regarding obesity, not solely due to the pervasive rhetoric about the "risks" associated with fat bodies, but because of the perception that these bodies represented markers of Indianness and facilitated social connections among Indians, standing in stark contrast to thinner bodies, which often symbolize whiteness. It would be simplistic to categorize these communities merely by their conditions, ignoring the multifaceted narratives woven into their experiences as they are often portrayed—whether as obese, unhealthy, impoverished, or just "bad at life" (Belcourt 2018). Some public health and biomedical discourses are just not fully up for making sense of obesity and diabetes in Indian communities, affixing these diseases to indigeneity in a broader public health imaginary. Throughout this work, I was continuously reminded of Belcourt's (2018:2) claim, "colonial affects escape analytic capture," recalling his words about how simple it could be to think that the reservation is bad *for* life because its members are bad *at* life. Yet, amidst the significant suffering and challenges, there exists an extraordinary resilience, a resistance, a refusal to die, and an embrace of creative and vital modes of living, making-do, and just *being* that nurture potential and possibility for better lives, better worlds, and better futures. It is my hope that this project illustrates how Indigenous women in the Choctaw Nation actively resist reductive interpretations that equate conditions such as obesity and diabetes with lives lived poorly—the culprits of COVID run loose in Indian bodies—and thus challenge simplistic narratives of individual blame and trauma within Indigenous communities—certainly during the COVID-19 pandemic, but also in the day-to-day.

In exploring the food-centered life histories shared by these women who recounted their lived experiences of life on the reservation, a recurring theme emerged: the recollection of past traumatic events that serves both as a public narrative and personal experience, enabling them to contextualize and make sense of their contemporary realities. These are lived realities characterized by interrupted traditions and reimagined Choctaw culture expressed in everyday life. It is within particular experiences of struggle, poverty, and discrimination—"an exhausted existence of indigeneity"—that historical trauma serves as a powerful and useful conceptual matrix, a starting point for meaning-making. Specific to obesity, historical trauma emerges as a foundational force that shapes all other contributing factors. The presence of obesogenic environments is directly tied to centuries of colonization and assimilation policies that displaced Indigenous peoples from their lands and stripped them of the resources necessary to lead self-determined lives. Historical and ongoing policies—such as boarding schools, forced removals, restrictions on fishing and hunting, and water access limitations—have resulted in impoverished food landscapes and the erosion of traditional knowledge systems, disrupting intergenerational transmission of foodways and survival skills. As a result, "commod bods" are not merely risk factors for COVID-19; they are the embodied consequences of biocultural trauma, inseparable from indigeneity's racialized terrain. "Commod bods," "COVID bods"— these identities are shaped by histories of structural violence and are situated within the biocultural, where disease and racialization intersect. More specifically, fat bodies, particularly those shaped by commodity foods and further impacted by COVID-19, become co-constitutive with indigeneity in an era where health is wielded as a biopolitical metric— one that measures the extent to which individuals can biologically and psychologically adapt to systemic oppression (Belcourt 2018).

During the pandemic, the Choctaw Nation's monthly news publication chronicled narratives of both loss and perseverance within the tribe. Featured in the July 2021 *Biskinik* was the story of beloved elders and highly respected knowledge holders Jerry and Shirley Lowman.[2] They both grew up in the rural hills speaking only *Chahta anumpa* until grade school, met in high school, and married soon thereafter. Their lifelong partnership was rooted in Choctaw heritage—music, dance, art, and language— and community. During the height of the pandemic, they were diligent in their efforts to protect themselves from COVID: They minimized their outings, stayed home, and were very careful around others during the outbreak. However, a knee injury forced Jerry into an unexpected visit to the emergency room, which then required a transfer to an out-of-state hospital for surgery. Due to visitor restrictions at the hospital during COVID, Shirley was unable to visit Jerry throughout his recovery. Once she could though, both Shirley and Jerry contracted COVID, which also spread to other family members. Shirley and Jerry were admitted to the same hospital at the same time, and tragically they both succumbed to the virus within eight days of each other, each unaware of the other's passing. Their family alone lost several dozens of people. Tammie Dugger, an emergency room nurse at the Choctaw Nation Health Center in Talihina, was quoted reflecting on the unpredictable nature of COVID's impact: "We were having to send people to Denver, to St. Louis, to Washington, because there were no beds available. We'd never seen stats that low before. You would have a very healthy person, and they would be the one who passed away. And then you would have a person with comorbidities, and they would survive. There has been no rhyme or reason on who survived and who did not survive this."

What if we pause here, on ER nurse Tammie's reflection that sometimes seemingly healthy people die while those with comorbidities survive? This paradox offers a point of departure for rethinking the conditions that shape survival, for understanding modes of being that protect bodies and lives and invite deeper inquiry into the social and relational factors that offer protection (or that leave bodies and lives vulnerable). Rather than reducing health outcomes to biomedical determinism, this perspective allows for survival to be contingent on more than individual physiology, but to also include the collective, the relational, and the structural. Women's stories reveal that food operates in multiple registers: The very commodities implicated in the creation of "commod bods"— foods framed as risk factors, that injure bodies, and that are linked to increased vulnerability to COVID-19—are also transformed into sources of nourishment and survival. When extra foods from the Food Distribution stores are repurposed into care packages for neighbors, elders, and those in need, these foods become more than mere sustenance. They become conduits of kinship, acts of reciprocity, and affirmations of Choctaw communal responsibility. In this way, the paradox of survival extends beyond biomedical explanations and into the realm of social meaning. Health is not simply an individual state but a deeply embedded, relational process shaped by historical dispossession and contemporary resilience. The very foods that signify loss and dependency (commodity foods) also sustain networks of care, forming a resistance to the logic of settler colonial elimination. This dialectic—where that which harms can also heal, where the imposed can become the reclaimed—underscores a Choctaw framework of interdependence, where survival is a collective act, bound by histories of endurance and the radical possibilities of community care.

In response to the pandemic, tribes in Oklahoma, including the Choctaw Nation, emerged as leaders in providing organized and accessible vaccination and treatment—not just for their own citizens but for the broader communities across the state of Oklahoma. In a time when federal and state responses faltered or proved inadequate, tribal nations stepped in, demonstrating a sovereignty rooted not only in governance but in the deeply held Indigenous values of caretaking, reciprocity, and collective responsibility. This act of widespread care serves as a powerful counterpoint to the narrative of Indigenous communities as vulnerable, passive recipients of aid; instead, it reaffirms the ways in which Indigenous nations have long been at the forefront of mutual aid and survival strategies, even—or especially—when faced with ongoing social abandonment. This response also challenges the idea that "commod bods" and "COVID bods" represent inevitable, predetermined fates. As Belcourt (2018) reminds us, settler colonialism is not an irreversible structure; it is reparable, and Indigenous peoples continue to enact radical refusals against the systems that seek to erase them. The Choctaw Nation's public health response stands as an example of what is possible when health is understood beyond individual pathology and risk factors, and instead as a condition shaped by structural inequalities, historical trauma, ongoing political realities, and how people make sense of these experiences.

However, it is essential to recognize the complexities and limitations of applying an embodied heritage framework universally, even within Indigenous communities across the United States. The ways in which historical trauma, violence, and social inequities shape lived experiences are deeply specific to each tribal nation, influenced by distinct histories, geographies, and cultural contexts. While an embodied heritage framework offers a valuable lens for understanding obesity among Choctaws in Oklahoma—particularly for those reliant on government commodity foods—the nuances of how these narratives unfold in different Indigenous communities must be carefully considered. First, the ways individuals and communities make meaning of their experiences and construct public narratives are shaped by subtle yet significant distinctions in historical and social positioning. These differences must be examined rather than assumed to be uniform across Indigenous populations. Second, there are major variations in how structural inequalities manifest. For instance, in urban areas such as Tulsa or Oklahoma City, where the commodity foods program does not extend, Natives in need might turn to food banks. This form of food dependency may not carry the same cultural significance or historical continuity as it does for reservation Natives who have a long relationship with government-issued commodities. While urban Natives may still associate food insecurity with broader colonial legacies, the absence of explicitly "Indian" foods (i.e., USDA-stamped commodity foods) in these systems alters how food dependency is tied to indigeneity and collective memory. Furthermore, the stigma attached to food banks and pantries in urban spaces differs from the normalized, historical reliance on commodity foods in rural communities, affecting how individuals negotiate their relationship with government food aid.

Despite these variations, the broader historical, political-economic, and social inequities that persist among Oklahoma's Native communities remain central to the embodied heritage framework. While the framework may require adaptation to account for community-specific differences, its core argument—that health is contingent on social, economic, historical, cultural, and political position *and* the structures of meaning that make sense of this experience—remains deeply relevant.

The embodied heritage framework offers valuable insight into the future of health and well-being among Indigenous peoples, aligning with what Kirmayer and colleagues (2014:309) describe as serving "the emancipatory goals of Indigenous decolonization." In calling attention to historical trauma and contemporary forms of violence, it simultaneously highlights the resilience, strength, and continuity of Indigenous communities, attending to both resistance and survival, trauma and renewal—an interplay that is evident across Indigenous communities in the United States and beyond. For example, as I described in the introduction, the political-economic and social conditions that contribute to high rates of obesity include "food deserts," referring to limited or nonexistent access to affordable, high-quality fresh food. However, food advocates and recent studies (Cummins et al. 2014; Dubowitz et al. 2015; USDA ERS 2016) argue that supermarket proximity is only one factor influencing food choices, while neighborhood resources, education, and cultural food preferences are often more decisive. Additionally, activists criticize the term "food desert" as an outsider's perspective that overlooks the agency, vibrancy, and potential of these communities (Brones 2018). Urban food activist Karen Washington instead advocates for the term *food apartheid*, which considers the entire food system, encompassing race, geography, faith, and economic inequalities (Brones 2018). This shift in language reframes food insecurity as a structural injustice rather than an environmental inevitability, opening space for deeper conversations about trauma, violence, heritage, and identity.

For Indigenous communities, the concept of *food apartheid* is closely tied to the broader movement for *food sovereignty*, a term originating from Central and South American Indigenous movements advocating for the right to land, territories, natural resources, and cultural practices, including language and food traditions (United Nations Declaration of Atitlán, accessed July 18, 2016). Food sovereignty aligns with the embodied heritage framework by drawing attention to the external forces that have long threatened Indigenous food systems and bodies, reinforcing the idea that struggles for rights—whether fishing, hunting, or water rights—are not simply about access but about cultural survival. These fights, many of which date back to the Trail of Tears, must be understood as early assertions of food sovereignty and identity, framed within tribal sovereignty and treaty rights. For Choctaws, this means reclaiming and protecting "first foods," which include deer, pokeweed, sumpweed seeds, hickory nuts, and greenbriar roots, among others. These foods are more than sustenance; they are living connections to land, history, and cultural knowledge. The struggle for their protection is not just a contemporary issue but a continuation of a long history of resisting colonial dispossession and cultural erasure. In this way, food sovereignty is a crucial dimension of embodied heritage, affirming that Indigenous health is inseparable from history, identity, and the right to self-determined futures.

In 2017, the Choctaw Nation partnered with Oklahoma State University's (OSU) Center for Sovereign Nations and OSU researchers to launch an heirloom crops initiative, the Growing Hope Program. Funded by the USDA, the project established a greenhouse at the capitol in Tuskahoma to study the cultivation, production, nutritional value, and potential commercialization of heirloom crops (Thompson et al. 2023). Among the varieties cultivated were dry beans, hominy corn, flower corn, squash, tobacco, lamb's-quarter, and a field pea variety originating from Mississippi. For Maudell Meshaya, a Choctaw tribal citizen, the project became an opportunity to revive a family legacy. She contributed a handful of Choctaw bean seeds—just nine in total—preserved through generations, with the hope that they would flourish in the greenhouse. "It came down from my grandfather, who gardened a lot. He grew everything. He had those beans, and he passed them on to my grandmother, then my mother, and then to me," she recalled. "I was able to grow them in the 1970s, so to carry it on would be wonderful." Edmond Perkins, a lifelong farmer within the Choctaw Nation, planted *tanchi* corn along the garden plot beside his home. The results were astonishing. "We planted it, and it got up tall. It got taller and taller and wound up fifteen feet tall, which is amazing. It had huge brace roots coming down," he shared. "The corn is really good tasting. It's good for you, full of vitamins. It's basically history, the flavor of history." For the first time in four generations, a small group of Choctaw elders gathered to share a meal of corn soup made from *tanchi* corn, an act that carried both nourishment and profound cultural meaning. As the elders reflected, the corn seeds had not just survived; they had remembered the land.

This act of reclamation—of planting, harvesting, and sharing traditional foods—is part of a broader movement of Choctaw survivance. Just as seeds hold the memory of the land, Choctaw bodies, stories, and practices remember history, making sense of the past in the present while shaping the future. The traumas of removal, dispossession, and cultural suppression live alongside acts of resilience and renewal. In this long process of decolonization, food becomes a bridge between generations, connecting ancestral knowledge to contemporary Choctaw lives. Today, through the Growing Hope Program, Choctaws across the United States can receive seeds and resources from the Choctaw Nation to cultivate their own healthy, sustainable, and culturally significant foods. In doing so, they are not only planting crops, but they are also planting history, memory, and a promise to future generations (Thompson et al. 2023).

To illustrate once more how an embodied heritage framework functions as an emancipatory force across time and space, I conclude with the story of *Ishtaboli* (stickball), a game deeply woven into Choctaw history and identity. Recognized as a precursor to modern lacrosse, *Ishtaboli* is one of the oldest organized sports in the United States. Its rules are simple yet physically demanding: Each player wields two *kapucha* (sticks) to maneuver the *towa* (ball) and attempts to strike the *fabvssa* (goal), a slender post approximately four inches in diameter and twelve feet tall. The game is played on a field comparable in size to an American football field, with teams of around thirty players engaging in an intense contest of skill, endurance, and strategy, where pushing, shoving, and tackling are integral to gameplay. Historically, *Ishtaboli* served as more than just a sport; it was a mechanism for conflict resolution, often replacing warfare as a means of settling disputes over land and resources. Today, it thrives within the Choctaw Nation as a powerful symbol of cultural resilience and renewal. The act of scoring in *Ishtaboli* is not just about winning a game; it reflects the broader pursuit of overcoming obstacles, a tangible reminder of the collective progress made in the face of adversity.

This metaphor extends beyond the playing field, speaking directly to contemporary struggles, including health disparities like obesity. Within *Ishtaboli*, there exists a nurturing space where Choctaw youth, regardless of athletic background, can develop confidence, perseverance, and a sense of belonging. The game teaches more than physical agility; it fosters discipline, collaboration, and endurance helpful for navigating life's challenges. Through stickball, players learn that success is not just individual but collective, grounded in relationships and shared effort. So, more than just a sport, *Ishtaboli* functions as a living narrative, an embodiment of Choctaw survivance, and the assertion of Indigenous presence, identity, and resilience despite ongoing colonial forces. Joey Tom, now a tribal councilmember, eloquently explained to me that *Ishtaboli* is not confined to the field; it is a philosophy for life, a way of understanding challenges and choices. He described how the game mirrors our journey through life, where obstacles (i.e., opposing players attempting to tackle) represent hardships that must be navigated with skill, adaptability, and determination. To reach the goal, one must stay focused, make quick decisions, and keep moving forward, just as in life:

> Stickball is a way of healing. You can look at it either way you want to. You can look at it like, if you're in trouble . . . the object of the game is to score, alright? You at least gotta have a goal, which that's our goal. You've got to score. That's our goal. So in life, you've got to have a goal in life, too. There's going be a lot of barriers that are going to be holding you down. There's going to be things—and if those defenders are coming after you, fixing

to tackle you, those are ways you can use that. . . . You make the wrong choices, your life's going to fall. You're gonna take the bad road. So, if you make the wrong decision, you're going to get tackled. But if you make the right decision, you move a different way, you try juking[3] or anything like that, you go to the next one. . . . And if you choose to stay positive, you'll make the right decision, and he won't be able to tackle you, he won't be able to make fun of you, or things like that. But by the time you reach the goal, you have touched the goal with your sticks, or you have a shot and made it from there, you turn around look behind you, and you see all those guys behind you. The whole concept of the game was the score, but you look at it and look at the things that you've had to get away from, that's back behind you. You can use stickball in that way. That's what we do, we use stickball. You can use it in different ways. You can use it in life situations. . . . That's how we tell our story about it. (Joey Tom, Durant)

Through this lens, *Ishtaboli* is more than a game—it is a mode of healing, a continuation of Choctaw identity, and a guide for thriving in a world that has long sought to erase Indigenous ways of knowing and being. In its rhythm, its movement, and its strategy, it carries the past into the present, offering a pathway for Choctaws to reclaim history, find strength in community, and envision a future shaped by resilience and self-determination.

NOTES

INTRODUCTION

1. Chilocco was one of five non-reservation boarding schools authorized by Congress in 1882. The other four non-reservation boarding schools include Carlisle Indian Industrial School in Pennsylvania, Haskell Indian Nations University in Kansas, Chemawa Indian School in Oregon, and Fort Simcoe in Washington state.

2. "Annie" refers to Aunt Irene, my grandmother's older sister, my great-aunt. It's an affectionate derivative of "Auntie" that my dad created when he was a child. As affectionate nicknames generally stick, everyone called her "Annie" for the rest of her life, her real name forgotten by some. This is one way family stories cannot be traced.

3. Pokni and Annie were the granddaughters of Chief Jefferson Gardner. Their family was well known, respected, financially comfortable, and cultivated peanuts on a significant amount of land in the area. According to my dad, this is how the town of Durant, Oklahoma, came to be known, for a short time, as "the peanut capital of the world."

4. This was surprising because statistics for American Indians are notoriously difficult to find, and few people outside of public health work speak about statistics. This indicated to me how the language of public health, probably through the various obesity initiatives in these communities, has circulated among these communities.

5. Adding a historical perspective, the allotment era that broke up collective land into individual tracts allotted to enrolled tribal peoples is a fundamental piece of structural violence that led to these experiences.

6. The NHANES is the source of the national obesity data cited here. The two main advantages of NHANES data are that it examines a nationally representa-

tive sample of Americans aged two years and older, and it combines interviews with physical examinations. The disadvantages of the survey are that it takes time from collection to reporting and that the survey size is small (about five thousand interviews) and is not designed for state or local data use. For state and local data, the Behavioral Risk Factor Surveillance System (BRFSS) is employed. Advantages of the BRFSS are three-fold: (1) It is the largest ongoing telephone health survey in the world, with an estimated 450,000 interviews annually; (2) each state survey is representative of the population of that state; and (3) BRFSS is conducted annually, so new obesity data are available each year. However, there are two major limitations of BRFSS: (1) It uses self-reported weight and height, which results in an underestimate of obesity rates due to people's tendency to over-report their height and under-report their weight; and (2) sample sizes in some states are too small to be useful for providing estimates about racial and ethnic groups. Thus, American Indians and Alaska Natives (AI/ANs) are often left out of all obesity reports.

7. I use the term AI/AN specifically in this section because the majority of public health research classifies Native peoples using this term. Throughout the book, I interchange the words Native American, Native, American Indian, Indian, Indigenous, Choctaw, or Chahta when referring to Indigenous peoples in this project. This is reflective of how people talk about themselves, often using multiple ways to refer to indigeneity.

8. The state also ranks fiftieth for fruit consumption nationally: More than half of AI adults (55 percent) report not eating even a single piece of fruit daily (OSDH 2022).

9. This number seemed impressively high to me, so I checked the program's eligibility requirements. The program is free and open to the public and does not require citizenship, membership, or connection to any tribe or tribal nation. In other words, anyone living within the CNO service area is eligible to become a member. Anyone over seventy-five years old (and their spouse) who lives outside the CNO is also eligible to become a member. The CNO will provide the registration fee for a designated number of selected walks/runs/events throughout the year, so it is an attractive program for anyone interested in walks/runs or wanting to get involved in walks/runs (CNO 2025).

10. The socio-demographic risk factors for food insecurity in Indigenous populations include poverty, multi-child households, low levels of education achievement and employment, reliance on social services (e.g., welfare or government subsidies), and single-parent households (Che and Chen 2011; Willows et al. 2012).

11. For reference, the national average food insecurity rate was 12 percent in 2016 (USDA ERS 2016).

12. Summers are notoriously very hot; there is rarely an autumn (weather seems to go from hot to cold, with no in-between); winters are unpredictable and can be freezing or warm; and spring marks tornado season and flooding.

13. All names are pseudonyms to protect the privacy of the participants in this project.

CHAPTER 1

1. *Humma* is spelled various ways, sometimes with an *o* or *u* as the second letter and sometimes with a single or double *m*. Some *Chahta anumpa* speakers are critical of a simplistic translation, however, arguing that *humma*, when applied to people, is an honorific that refers to brave, courageous, or honorable. In this translation, "Oklahoma" means an honorable people, brave people, or courageous people.

   Following the tumultuous period of the Civil War, representatives from the Five Civilized Tribes, including the Choctaw Nation, journeyed to Washington, D.C. Their mission was to reestablish formal ties with the U.S. government, which had been strained due to the events surrounding the war. During these discussions, the concept of an Indian Territory was proposed by federal officials. Choctaw delegate Rev. Allen Wright suggested an impactful name for this proposed territory: *Oklahumma* (*Biskinik* 2010; Meserve 1941:319). Hence, the term *Oklahumma* could be translated as "Red People's Territory" or, in the context of its proposed use, the Oklahoma Territory. Today, the name "Oklahoma" persists, and, translated literally, "the State of Oklahoma" means "the State Belonging to Red People" (*Biskinik* 2010).

2. The term *removal* inadequately describes the forced expulsion of Native Americans, which was far more violent than the word suggests. Scholars argue that terms such as *ethnic cleansing* or *mass deportation* more accurately reflect the brutality of these events (Banner 2005; Carson 2008; Saunt 2020; Snyder 2017). Far from a single act, Indian removal was a prolonged series of betrayals reshaping North America (Snyder 2017). It was central to the Jacksonian era, deeply tied to economic shifts and the expansion of slavery, and contributing to tensions that led to the Civil War (Hanson 2021; Snyder 2017).

3. All U.S. Census data is based on self-reported information. Since 2000, the Census has allowed individuals to identify with more than one racial category. Those who select both American Indian or Alaska Native along with other racial identities are categorized as "American Indian or Alaska Native in combination." In contrast, individuals who select only American Indian or Alaska Native are classified as "American Indian or Alaska Native alone."

   Among U.S. states, Oklahoma has the highest proportion of individuals identifying as American Indian alone, followed by Arizona (13 percent), California (10 percent), New Mexico (9 percent), and Texas (5 percent) (U.S. Census Bureau 2020).

   The Navajo Nation represents the largest portion of the American Indian alone population at 15 percent, with the Cherokee Nation following at 10 percent. The Choctaw Nation is the third largest at 3 percent, followed by the Lumbee Tribe of North Carolina at just under 3 percent (U.S. Census Bureau 2020).

4. The United States currently acknowledges tribal nations as domestic dependent nations, placing tribes in a unique position between foreign nations and U.S. states, and defines the relationship between federal, state, and tribal governments through its legal system (DOJ 1995). There are currently 574 recognized tribal nations in the U.S., including 229 in Alaska. According to the National Congress of American Indians, Native peoples and governments possess inherent rights and maintain a political relationship with the U.S. government that is independent of race or ethnicity (NCAI 2018).

    Jimcy McGirt was convicted by an Oklahoma state court of three serious sexual offenses. It was later argued that the state lacked jurisdiction to prosecute McGirt because he is an enrolled member of the Seminole Nation, and the crimes occurred on Indian land, the Muscogee Creek Reservation. Under the Major Crimes Act (MCA), any Native American who commits certain offenses in Indian Country falls under the exclusive jurisdiction of the federal government, not the state. McGirt petitioned for a new trial in federal court, arguing that the Muscogee Creek Reservation had not been legally disestablished when Oklahoma became a state in 1907. In a landmark decision on July 9, 2020, Justice Neil Gorsuch affirmed that, for the purposes of the MCA, land reserved for the Muscogee Creek Nation since the nineteenth century remains Indian Country. This decision was based on a treaty from 1833 that guaranteed the Muscogee Creek Nation a permanent homeland "as long as they shall exist as a nation and continue to occupy the country." Similarly, the Treaty of Dancing Rabbit Creek (1830) provided the Choctaw Nation assurances that their land would remain theirs "while they shall exist as a Nation and live on it," with the United States pledging to protect it from incorporation into any state or territory. The Supreme Court's ruling in *McGirt v. Oklahoma* affirmed the continued existence of the Muscogee Creek Reservation, setting a precedent that other reservations established through historic treaties were never legally dissolved upon Oklahoma's statehood. This decision has had profound implications for the Choctaw Nation, reinforcing its sovereign status and shaping its legal framework, governance, and relationships with both the State of Oklahoma and neighboring communities.

5. Traditionally, the Choctaw Nation has referred to "ten-and-a-half counties" as its jurisdiction or geographic boundaries, as this area is most commonly used for determining eligibility for tribal services and programs. However, due to the *McGirt v. Oklahoma* decision, the "ten-and-a-half counties" designation no longer aligns with the current geography or jurisdiction of the Choctaw reservation. The reservation's boundaries have reverted to those established by the Treaty of Dancing Rabbit Creek. Despite this change, the Choctaw Nation continues to use the term "ten-and-a-half counties" to determine eligibility for programs and services.

6. Freedmen descendants continue to advocate for tribal citizenship, drawing parallels to broader racial justice movements in the United States. The Cherokee

Nation's 2017 decision to reinstate Freedmen rights has increased pressure on the Choctaw Nation (and others) to follow suit. However, these tribes maintain that their sovereignty grants them the right to set their own membership criteria, even as critics argue that such exclusions contradict the fundamental principles of tribal self-determination and historical accountability. Roberts (2021) and Waldman (2023) suggest that reconciliation between Freedmen and tribal nations will require not just legal battles but also a broader shift in how sovereignty is understood and applied. If sovereignty is to serve as a mechanism for justice and self-determination, it must also reckon with the historical exclusions that continue to shape the lived experiences of Freedmen descendants.

7.   Tribal service areas include tribal lands and nearby areas outside their boundaries; they are the geographic areas in which federal or tribal programs have responsibilities.

8.   The seven states smaller than the Choctaw reservation are Massachusetts, Vermont, New Hampshire, New Jersey, Connecticut, Delaware, and Rhode Island.

9.   Across the state of Oklahoma, there are thirty-nine federally recognized tribes; only five are considered indigenous to Oklahoma: Osage, Caddo, Kiowa, Comanche, and Wichita.

10. Recognizing this legacy challenges simplistic narratives of historical trauma and raises important questions about how historical trauma is remembered and whose histories are centered.

11. Reba McEntire was born in McAlester, OK and raised on a ranch in a small town near Atoka. She continues to have ties to southeastern Oklahoma, with family still living and working in the area.

12. Based on CNO in-house research that includes license plate surveys, sign-in sheets, regular and periodic visitor interviews, and surveys conducted to determine visitor origins for the resort. This information was provided to me during an interview with a participant who had worked at the resort.

13. The state receives a share of revenues from tribes in exchange for exclusive gaming rights. Across tribes in the state with gaming revenue, this amounts to approximately $150 million annually, with most of the money going to Oklahoma schools.

14. In 2021, the Cherokee and Choctaw Nations announced that they would begin issuing their own hunting licenses to tribal citizens. This decision followed Oklahoma Governor Kevin Stitt's refusal to renew the state's existing hunting and fishing license agreements with the tribes. The dispute is the latest in a series of tensions between the tribes and Stitt dating back to 2019, when the governor attempted to renegotiate gaming compacts. These tensions were further heightened by the *McGirt v. Oklahoma* Supreme Court decision, which Stitt has repeatedly opposed.

     Governor Stitt has argued that all Oklahomans should be treated equally under the law, citing this as a reason for not renewing the hunting compacts.

Former Governor Mary Fallin negotiated with the tribes in 2015 and 2016, whereby the tribes agreed to buy a collective minimum of 200,000 licenses every year for $2 each, plus pay administrative fees. In addition to those payments, the state received more federal grants that are determined in part by license sales. The two tribes' purchases accounted for almost 20 percent of sales in 2021. *Minko* ("Chief") Gary Batton stated, "The reality is we did not have to pay anything, and that's the path we're going down," as both Cherokee and Choctaw chiefs rejected the proposal, asserting their nations' treaty rights and emphasizing their sovereignty (Young 2021). Both tribes now allow citizens to hunt under their own tribal laws rather than state regulations, signaling a shift from state-based to treaty-based governance.

15. The trauma of forced removal, land dispossession, and cultural loss is a central theme in discussions of Indigenous historical memory. However, as Roberts (2021) argues, historical trauma within Indigenous nations must also include recognition of how the institution of slavery shaped Choctaw society and its aftermath. The descendants of enslaved people have their own histories of forced migration, racial discrimination, and disenfranchisement that parallel and intersect with Indigenous experiences of colonization. By including Freedmen in the history of Choctaw removal and settlement in Indian Territory, scholars can more fully account for the multifaceted ways in which racial hierarchies and colonial policies shaped Indigenous nations and their relationships to Black communities.

16. After the Civil War, Choctaw Freedmen were largely excluded from the economic opportunities granted to tribal citizens, despite their historical ties to the Nation. U.S. treaty obligations promised them certain rights, but access to land, resources, and economic mobility was systematically denied. The Dawes Act and allotment policies further marginalized Freedmen, leaving many landless and pushing them into economic precarity while reinforcing racial divisions within Indigenous communities (Krauthamer 2013).

17. Historically, tribes have been recognized as sovereign entities only in specific situations, such as when state governments try to enforce regulations within tribal lands. The Supreme Court has affirmed that the federal Indian trust responsibility entails upholding the highest "moral obligations" to safeguard tribal rights. This trust duty holds considerable importance in federal administrative decisions and can be enforced in court as a fiduciary responsibility (Calabrese 2024).

18. Throughout each interview, I noted the themes addressed, which allowed me to shape each interview to the participant's style and at the same time ensure that my questions were answered. Some women needed a great deal of prompting, but once the broad questions were answered, the majority of women needed only slight probing to address the questions at the heart of this study. Themes around identity emerged mostly around memories of food experiences growing up, which also prompted most participants to discuss historical trauma and life challenges.

19. The surveys used included the Medical Outcomes Study Short-Form Survey (SF-36), the Gustafson Perceived Food Environment Measure (GPFEM); the Native American Acculturation Scale (NAAS); the Historical Losses Scale (HLS); and the Body Image Assessment for Obesity (BIA-O). I selected these instruments based on their validity and reliability, as well as their usage with Native peoples (the NAAS and HLS were specifically developed in consultation with Native communities). However, I remained aware all along that any instrument is both incomplete and insufficient without the ethnographic understanding that helps me makes sense of how these tools in turn make sense of the issues.

20. To limit geographical bias in the sample, participants were recruited from five sites: Broken Bow, Durant, McAlester, Poteau, and Talihina.

The length of time required for the interview varied based on the length of time individuals took to process and respond to each question (e.g., some women responded directly to each question, while others wanted to discuss the meaning of each question and response) and on the emotional output in response to the questions, particularly in response to emotional questions in the qualitative interview and historical losses inventory.

I had the great fortune to work with incredible staff at the Food Distribution stores and community centers, who were more than accommodating of my research. The director of the Food Distribution Program in the Nation, Jerry Tonubbee, was integral to the success of this research, offering his personal office as space for the interviews and coordinating tours of the locations and space for participant observation.

21. Women were compensated $50 for their time for the food-centered life history interview, which likely functioned as an incentive for participation as well. This rate was decided because participation in the interview and completion of the quantitative instruments was time-intensive and burdensome.

22. The study was advertised in the Choctaw newspaper and on posters at the Food Distribution stores, community centers, and Indian churches; information was also emailed to all Choctaw employees. However, most participants were recruited on-site or were referred by other participants.

23. Other reported tribal affiliations included Cherokee, Creek, Chickasaw, and Shoshone.

CHAPTER 2

1. The Kiamichi Mountains, a subrange of the Ouachita Mountains, is the namesake of Kiamichi Country, the official tourism designation for southeastern Oklahoma.

2. This is an interesting comment to me because this television show is famous not necessarily (although sometimes) for obscure ingredients, but rather for the unusual combinations of ingredients which are often not commonly prepared together. For example, in the episode "Yucca, Watermelon, Tortillas,"

ingredients for the appetizer portion consisted of watermelon, canned sardines, pepper jack cheese, and zucchini. What I find most interesting is that Linda goes on to describe the fast-food chains she frequents and the foods she eats, which have ingredients that are truly unknown. I can't help but recall Michael Pollan's (2008) widely quoted mantra: "If you can't pronounce it, don't eat it," and I wonder if Linda is also aware of it. Even more importantly, I wonder how this mantra means different things to different people who have varying degrees of food security.

3. At 5'4", Linda weighs 232 pounds and has a waist circumference of 54 inches. Though the body mass index is not a reliable and appropriate measurement for individuals, her BMI is 39.9, which positions her in the severely obese category. I collected these data for all participants as part of the larger project but offer them here as descriptive tools.

4. Linda's reference to diabetes as "just statistics" is a striking example of how public health narratives become internalized. The disease is not only a biological condition but also a marker of historical and structural violence. By categorizing diabetes as an inevitable, hereditary part of being Indigenous, she reflects a fatalistic worldview that blurs the lines between individual agency and systemic forces. This is meaning-making at its most painful: Chronic illness is seen as both a personal burden and an inescapable cultural legacy.

5. The comfort food Linda is referring to includes potato chips, Kool-Aid jammers, Little Debbie packaged pastries, and candies of all sorts. None of these foods is available through the commodities foods program.

6. Certificate of Degree of Indian Blood (CDIB) is a document issued by the Bureau of Indian Affairs (BIA) that specifies an individual's blood quantum and tribal affiliation. The CDIB is controversial due to its connection to racial politics, eugenics, and because non-federally recognized tribes and certain groups, like Freedmen, are ineligible. Blood quantum is a colonial concept developed to measure the proportion of "Native blood" a person possesses, expressed as a fraction based on family lineage. It is rooted in pseudo-scientific ideas and lacks biological validity—human inheritance doesn't work in fixed ratios that can accurately "measure" someone's Native ancestry. The concept was implemented by the U.S. government, primarily to weaken Native sovereignty and dispossess Indigenous people from their lands, resources, and culture. In 1884, the BIA used Census rolls to assign blood quantum values to Natives, often with inaccuracies. Linda's statement captures the contested nature of Indigenous identities. Official documents and bureaucratic categories attempt to simplify and divide, but Linda's personal identity resists these neat classifications. Her identification as "full-blood" reflects both a reclaiming of knowledge and a protest against limitations imposed by state systems—a subtle form of resistance to the structural violence that has long sought to define and contain Native identities.

7. This brief mention touches on the legacy of land allotment policies and the later development of Indian housing programs. The decision not to take up available support or the ambiguous reasons behind it can be read as a marker of mistrust in state and federal systems, an understandable response given a history of broken promises and disenfranchisement.

8. *Everyday violence* (Scheper-Hughes 1993) refers to the normalized, routine abuses—both physical and emotional—that individuals endure. In Linda's recounting of her childhood, violence was a familiar part of daily life. Her retrospective view points to an evolving understanding of what constitutes abuse. As a kid, this kind of treatment was normalized, reflecting the cycle of violence that can be internalized in communities facing broader structural neglect. This normalization of violence is a survival mechanism but also a painful reminder of how abuse is woven into the fabric of daily existence for many Indigenous women and children.

9. Although now framed in the narrative as part of her past, the violence was a normalized part of caregiving and familial relationships. This everyday violence is both literal (physical abuse) and metaphorical: It speaks to the way that care and punishment were inextricably linked in a context of lack of resources, collectivity, and generational trauma. Telling this story about her mother, Linda links this memory with her own self-described pickiness around eggs that she shared at the beginning of the interview. Although we don't discuss it, the look of surprise at this connection is written all over her face and can be heard in her voice.

10. Although Linda herself has only fragmented memories of her mother's boarding school experience, this forced removal from her cultural context is a clear instance of historical trauma. The boarding school system was designed to erase Indigenous identities—a form of structural violence that disrupted family structures and cultural continuity. Linda's silence about the details, "I don't know nothing about [my parents]," underscores the lasting impact of that trauma, as generations struggle with an interrupted lineage of knowledge and identity.

11. This passage speaks directly to structural violence—the policies and systems that left Linda and her family with inadequate housing, utilities, and opportunities. The reference to "dirt poor" conditions, lack of electricity, and running water isn't merely an economic statement; it reflects the historical dispossession and marginalization of Native communities. This systemic neglect is a direct product of federal policies that aimed to undermine Indigenous ways of life, contributing to the violence and trauma that still shapes Linda's life.

12. In this passage, Linda negotiates between individual responsibility and a broader, almost predetermined, cultural fate. The intertwining of religious fatalism ("the good Lord's will") with medical determinism reveals the complex meaning-making processes that arise in contexts where personal choices are

constrained by historical and structural violence. Her struggle to reconcile these influences underscores how health is both a personal and communal narrative, reflective of deep-seated historical trauma.

13. *Symbolic violence* is the internalized devaluation and stigmatization that comes from pervasive negative stereotypes and cultural erasure. It often manifests in how people talk about themselves and their communities, reinforcing a sense of inferiority. These remarks expose the symbolic violence of cultural stereotyping. Linda recounts how others reduce Choctaws to drunkenness, an image that is as reductive as it is damaging. By repeating this stereotype—even with a chuckle—she demonstrates how pervasive and normalized these discourses have become. It's a reminder that the label "Native" carries not just historical trauma, but ongoing cultural devaluation in the public sphere.

14. Here, Linda was correlating loss of *Chahta anumpa* with alcoholism and diabetes.

15. The loss of language here is emblematic of violence and historical trauma. The erosion of *Chahta anumpa* is not just a loss of words but a loss of identity, history, cosmologies, and power. Linda's confusion over the language taught at the community center and what she remembers speaking (and how she currently speaks) highlights how even efforts at cultural reclamation can feel tainted if they do not align with the lived experiences and histories of community members. The trauma and violence are twofold: They come from external pressures to assimilate and from the internalized sense that one's knowledge and original teachings are somehow wrong.

16. The term *nahullo* is used colloquially for white person. It originates from stories about the *Oka Nahullo*, or the white beings of the water, who were believed to live in deep waters. They had light skin, often described as similar in color and texture to trout skins, and were believed to capture any human who looked them in the eye and convert them into a white water being like themselves.

17. Her BMI is 36; her waist circumference is 46.5 inches, measures which I offer for description only, aware of the problematic nature of the BMI. Her scores on the general health survey indicate that she is not limited physically, emotionally, or socially, nor does she report high pain. She scores low in the energy/fatigue domain, but as she reveals in the interview, that is because she is very active. She appears indeed to be in good health.

18. This passage reflects everyday violence in the form of a fatalistic attitude toward chronic disease. When diabetes becomes "just an Indian disease," it normalizes suffering and prevents proactive health behaviors. The acceptance of illness as inevitable can be seen as a consequence of historical and structural violence and neglect, where everyday living conditions and cultural messages combine to diminish both self-care and collective care—forms of violence that damage body and spirit.

19. Although Sherry herself did not attend boarding school, her friends' experiences evoke the legacy of assimilation policies designed to erase Indigenous

languages, practices, and identities. These forced assimilation practices not only harmed individuals at the time but continue to influence community self-esteem and identity and are relegated not only to boarding school experiences but to everyday settings like church. The pain of being "not allowed to be Indian" underscores how structural violence from state policies can reverberate across generations and across spaces.

20. This excerpt reveals interpersonal and institutional violence in a religious context. The exclusionary practices of white church members—separating Native congregants from the main body—illustrate everyday violence in the form of microaggressions and overt discrimination. It is a daily reminder of how Native peoples are treated as "Other" on their own reservations and even in spaces that claim universal equality, reinforcing feelings of marginalization and contributing to low self-esteem.

21. She is fully sobbing at this moment in the interview, but she tells me she wants to continue.

22. Sherry juxtaposes negative stereotypes with a strong affirmation of Choctaw spiritual depth. The disparaging remarks from outsiders (even those within church settings) represent symbolic violence, where negative images of Choctaw competence and identity are perpetuated. Yet, by asserting that Choctaws are more spiritual, Sherry reclaims her Choctaw heritage. This tension between external devaluation and internal affirmation is an ongoing part of meaning-making in Indigenous communities, illustrating how identity is continuously negotiated in the face of both historical trauma and everyday violence.

23. Right around the time of this interview with Sherry, the local news had covered a controversy about a large banner created by Oklahoma State University students for a football game against the Florida Seminoles. The banner read "Send 'em Home," followed by the hashtags used across social media, #Trail_of_Tears #GoPokes, to tag the images.

24. Sherry's shifting tone—from self-deprecating humor to critical commentary—reveals the struggle to reconcile personal responsibility with structural constraints. While she acknowledges the health consequences of lifestyle choices (such as eating habits fostered by cultural fellowship), she also points to systemic barriers like limited access to healthier food options. This dual framing is a form of meaning-making where health is both an individual choice and a reflection of broader social and economic conditions.

25. This reflection offers a window into what Sherry experiences as a very painful transformation of cultural practices and a dilution of Choctawness and Indianness, more broadly. Sherry's lament about losing the "Indian part" of the church and family life shows how assimilation pressures and intermarriage—fueled by both historical trauma and ongoing structural inequities—are reshaping what it means to be Choctaw. It is an expression of both loss and resistance: Even as the culture erodes, the desire to reclaim and celebrate being Choctaw remains strong.

26. Here, the poor quality of government-provided food speaks again to structural violence: The government's failure to provide nutritious, culturally appropriate food to Native families has long-lasting impacts on dietary habits and health. The experience of receiving old, bug-infested food is not only a reminder of poverty and neglect but also shows a serious lack of care or regard for Indian peoples, linking past injustices with present health disparities.

27. Sherry is referring to the license plates on cars. Tribal nations in Oklahoma have negotiated compacts with the state to provide partial reimbursement to tribal citizens for car registration and renewal fees.

28. Sherry's words here reflect symbolic violence, where a stigma attached to being Indian is internalized even within families. When Native identity is seen as something that must be "cashed in on" for benefits rather than celebrated as a heritage, it diminishes self-worth and perpetuates a cycle of shame. This internalized devaluation whereby her brother modifies his behavior and even denies parts of his identity to avoid discrimination hurts Sherry deeply.

29. Like Linda, Sherry's account of language loss illustrates symbolic violence as well. The dissonance between the "real" language of her grandmother and the standardized, modern version taught in class underscores how community members work to navigate a contested cultural space where authenticity is constantly questioned.

30. I intentionally use the word "misery" here, inspired by Belcourt's (2018:2) usage of the term in *Meditations on Reserve Life, Biosociality, and the Taste of Non-Sovereignty*. As Belcourt writes:

    Misery is a bad word. Harsh, even. But I think it is big enough to conceptualize the cramped conditions under which life is haphazardly improvised on the reserve. Misery wears you down, effecting both a corporeal fragility and an intellectual fatigue that double as sociality's background noise. I am recruiting misery here because it does not rest on the eventful. Instead, it blends into ordinary time. It is possible to make joy or to feel enlivened within a miserable context. But misery circumscribes the body's potentialities. If misery is a part of slow death's arsenal, if it hangs "in the air like a rumor," then there is no easy way out. Existence is what taxes.

31. Or, as we see in the Choctaw Nation's case, a restructuring, re-creation, or re-invention around cultural distinction that is in conversation with the goals and ambitions of the settler nation. I will return to this in-depth in chapter five.

32. For example, why do Choctaws no longer invite guests over? Why do folks no longer go to each other's homes? Is it in recognition that hosting is difficult and guests don't want to take away what little one has? Does it speak to lost systems of reciprocity, the "tyranny of the gift" (Mauss 1967); have Choctaw exchange systems around giving and receiving (reciprocity) been affected by commodity foods?

CHAPTER 3

1. For example, *collective trauma, intergenerational trauma, multi-generational trauma,* and *soul wound.*

2. Duran and Duran (1995:152) note, "The trauma of the loss of land, culture, and people has never been resolved, but has been anesthetized by alcohol and other drugs. Native American people suffer from post-traumatic stress disorder as a consequence of the devastating effects of genocide perpetrated by the U.S. government."

3. The findings from these studies linked an array of psychological problems among the children of Holocaust survivors with their parents' experiences, including symptoms of post-traumatic stress disorder (PTSD) and responses such as denial, depersonalization, isolation, memory loss, nightmares, hyper-vigilance, substance abuse, fixation on trauma, survivor guilt, and unresolved grief. For reviews of these studies, see, for example, Berger (1988), Ganz (2002), Rowland-Klein and Dunlop (1998), and Steinberg (1989).

4. E.g., African-American experiences of slavery; apartheid in South Africa; Cambodian experiences of Khmer Rouge; Hiroshima.

5. Namely, deaths due to increased morbidity and mortality rates, lowered life expectancy, and higher rates of accidental deaths.

6. E.g., unresolved grief, complicated/prolonged grief, PTSD, and depression.

7. Evans-Campbell (2008) attempted to address this problem by identifying three key characteristics of historical trauma events: 1) the event was widespread among a specific group or population, with many group members affected; 2) the event was perpetrated by out-group members with purposeful and often destructive intent; and 3) the event generated high levels of collective distress in the victimized group. Additionally, there seem to be generally agreed-upon characteristics of historical trauma responses, which comprise the following: 1) historical trauma events continue to undermine the wellbeing of contemporary group members; 2) responses to historical trauma events interact with contemporary stressors to influence wellbeing; and 3) the risk associated with historical trauma events can accumulate across generations (Bombay et al. 2014; Evans-Campbell 2008).

8. Sotero's (2006:99) conceptual model builds on the tenets of social epidemiology, specifically psychosocial theory, political-economic theory, and social-ecological systems theory (Krieger 2001; McMichael 1999) and posits that historical trauma originates with the "subjugation of a population by a dominant group" and requires the following four elements: 1) overwhelming physical and psychological violence; 2) segregation and/or displacement; 3) economic deprivation; and 4) cultural dispossession.

9. Sotero's (2006) model positions primary generations as the direct victims of subjugation and loss; plagued with physical, psychological, and emotional injuries; and trauma responses in line with PTSD, depression, and self-destructive behaviors. The model allows for a translation of psychological and emotional

disorders into physical disease and vice versa. Secondary (and subsequent) generations are affected by the original trauma through multiple means, e.g., impaired parenting capacity or impaired genetic functioning and expression that can be translated in utero or environmentally: Poor maternal care, malnutrition, and depressive state contribute to poor quality breast milk, low-birth weight babies, and fetal stress responses that are correlated with other negative health outcomes throughout life (e.g., Type 2 diabetes). Additionally, maladaptive behaviors and related social problems, including substance abuse, physical/sexual abuse, and suicide, directly traumatize offspring and are indirectly transmitted through learned behavior (i.e., the intergenerational cycle of trauma). "Vicarious traumatization," or the means by which traumatic events become embedded in the collective social memories through storytelling and oral traditions, may teach offspring to share in the ancestral pain and harbor strong feelings of unresolved grief. Second generations may also experience original trauma through loss of culture and language, as well as contemporary experiences of discrimination, injustice, poverty, and social inequality. These direct experiences may work to validate their knowledge of historical trauma. Finally, this model posits that the cumulative effects of historical trauma on the population result in a higher prevalence of social and physical ills that ultimately lead to population-specific health disparities.

10. Many Native and non-Native public health professionals have embraced this model (or variations of it) in efforts to develop intervention programs integrating historical trauma with community capacity and empowerment (e.g., Chino and DeBruyn 2006; Elias et al. 2012; Trinidad 2009; Willows et al. 2012).

11. This is problematic for at least two reasons. First, the adoption of clinical diagnoses underscores the denial of Indigenous means of dealing with trauma (Brave Heart 1995). Second, drawing from Gone and Kirmayer (2010), this seems best *not* approached at the pan-Indian (or macro level), because each Indigenous culture will have its own social and cultural methods for defining and resolving trauma (Kidron 2012). We must consider that conceptions of trauma are culturally defined and may not cross over from Indigenous communities to the clinical setting (Gone and Kirmayer 2010). McKinley (2012:227) writes, "Historical trauma, like all methodologies, is a product of its construction. With it, Duran and Duran and Brave Heart simultaneously blame colonization for the problems facing local Indigenous populations and create a methodology dependent upon Western clinical practise that is to be deployed on a pan-Indian level. In essence they conduct the same simplification of Indigenous peoples into 'Indians' that the colonial state's discourse does."

12. Maxwell notes that Indigenous healing providers draw from trauma discourse to legitimate individual and social suffering, as well as older therapeutic forms that center on sharing local social histories as a means to restore collective and cultural continuity and identity. She argues that historical trauma discourses invoked in these ways may work to continue the colonial discourse of mental

health and social welfare approaches that blamed Indigenous parenting practices for children's social problems and failure to assimilate.

13. They argue that analyzing and assessing attributions such as the cross-sectional correlation of familial attendance in boarding (residential) schools with mental health problems in later generations cannot disentangle past and present causal processes. Interpretive uncertainty will always remain even amid suggestive evidence linking exposure to violence in boarding schools with current problems, because mental health problems are common, multiply caused, and non-specific (Kirmayer et al. 2014:307).

14. For example, binaries of colonizer/colonized; victim/resilient; past/present; Western theory/Indigenous knowledge etc.

15. The United Nations Educational, Scientific, and Cultural Organization (UNESCO) is a specialized agency of the United Nations whose mission is to promote peace and security through international cooperation in education, the sciences, culture, and communication. Its key areas of focus include protecting cultural and natural heritage, promoting global literacy, supporting sustainable development, protecting press freedom and access to information, and preserving traditions and Indigenous knowledges.

16. One local high school eliminated Spanish and French and now offers only *Chahta anumpa* as a second language. Important to note, however, is that across high schools where *Chahta anumpa* is offered, it is an online course, meaning that students do not have an actual instructor but instead log into pre-recorded classes while sitting together in a classroom.

17. Lactose intolerance in exclusively breastfed infants is extremely rare. Breast milk is naturally rich in lactose, and most babies are born with the enzyme they need to digest it. True lactose intolerance in infancy—congenital lactase deficiency—is a very uncommon genetic condition that shows up right away with severe symptoms. More often, what gets labeled as *lactose intolerance* tends to be something else, like a temporary gut issue from an infection or a reaction to something in the mother's diet. So while digestive distress can definitely happen in breastfed babies, it's rarely caused by the lactose itself.

18. Nelly Coyote is, like all other names presented here, a pseudonym. I chose it deliberately because this participant's name is identifiably Native. For her middle name, her mother gave her an Indian name that was selected specifically for her. She went by her first name for most of her life until she became conscious of the American Indian Movement and felt "safe" to identify openly as Native. While living in New York City (NYC), she began to use her middle (Indian) name as her first name and was encouraged by friends to do so. She described, however, multiple instances in which her Indian name served as a source of embarrassment (her daughter asked her to not use it so she wouldn't be made fun of) or as a joke at her expense (one of her boyfriends teased her continuously, using her name as a platform to joke about Natives living in teepees and being backwards among friends in NYC). She mentioned that she wants to return to

using her first name because it is less identifiably Native. She is tired of being asked multiple questions about her name.

19. Nelly Coyote's father joined the army after finishing high school and was sent to war. Nelly Coyote notes, "When [dad] came back [from war], he was very religious. Mother said he wasn't before, but when he came back, he was a fanatic, and he was a preacher, and we moved around different churches all the time."

20. I ask Nelly how she ended up in NYC, and she tells me, "I had a friend in high school whose family was in the army, so she had been all over the world. . . . She brought me this magazine one time and it showed a picture of this woman running and jumping into the arms of a man in the Greenwich Village in New York, and there were streets—it was very romantic. . . . I told my friend, I said, "Well I'm going to go to New York City." And I did! I didn't even finish high school. I got on the Greyhound bus and went to New York City had $18 in my pocket. Without anyone. I had quite a life there for a while. Mostly I was with men. Different men, living with them. Gradually I learned how to live in the city and then I had one particular boyfriend, and I stayed with him four years. He's someone I traveled with. I made friends in college, you know, I just got older, and I was twenty-seven when I left." Nelly has visited multiple countries in Europe, Africa, and Asia, and repeatedly tells me about how beautiful she was when she was young, alluding that because she was so beautiful, many doors opened for her, including opportunities to travel the world (opportunities that were not available to her in Oklahoma or Texas).

21. Here, her voice breaks and she begins to cry, but she assures me that she wants to continue talking. The interview with Nelly is the longest interview in the project, lasting nearly five hours, as she shares so openly and freely with me, trusting me with her stories and words, and she says at the end that she has really enjoyed the experience; it felt healing to her. It felt healing to me too.

22. Here, Nelly Coyote is referring the purpose of the Indian boarding schools, which was to assimilate Indigenous children into Euro-American culture and "civilize" them by removing them from their families and communities and immersing them in English-language education, Christianity, and Euro-American cultural practices.

23. It seems as though Nelly Coyote perceives that her life—specifically the life she imagined and attempted to create for herself by running away to New York, Los Angeles, joining the Navy, etc.—was stolen from her before she was even born. *Stolen* in the sense that the trauma of her parents' experiences, her inherited trauma, set the parameters within which Nelly Coyote could thrive.

24. Red River Preparatory School is a pseudonym. The current tuition for high school at RRPS is $25,325 per year. In Oklahoma, this is a significant cost, and it is the most expensive school in the state. For reference, the average annual tuition for private high schools in Oklahoma is around $7,000, though this varies widely, as some schools provide financial aid programs that reduce the tuition to as low as $500.

CHAPTER 4

1   The Choctaw Princess and Royalty Program is a longstanding tradition that celebrates and cultivates strong, culturally grounded *Chahta ohoyo* ("Choctaw women"). Each year, local pageants are held in the twelve districts of the Choctaw Nation, where contestants are evaluated on their talent, poise, and traditional dress. One representative from each age division is selected to advance to the Choctaw Nation Royalty Pageant, held annually during the Labor Day festival at *Tvshka Homma*. There, three young women are crowned Little Miss, Junior Miss, and Miss Choctaw Nation. But the program is about much more than pageantry—it is a form of cultural preservation and leadership development. The pageant honors young women who embody and promote Choctaw values and traditions. During their one-year reign, royalty serve as ambassadors of the Choctaw Nation. They attend cultural classes, participate in community events, and represent the Nation with pride and dignity, helping to carry forward the language, customs, and spirit of the Choctaw people.

2.   The Choctaw Nation Color Guard was formed in 1998 for the purpose of honoring Choctaw veterans who have given their time in service to protect the United States. This group of Choctaw military veterans are widely esteemed, and they're often invited to post colors at tribal events and community organizations, render military funeral honors, lead grand entry at powwows, march in parades, and lead Trail of Tears commemorative walks.

3.   "That" refers to the Trail of Tears while "this" presumably refers to contemporary experiences of poverty, struggle, and discrimination.

4.   Wheelock Academy was cofounded by Alfred Wright, a physician and missionary who, along with his wife, traveled with Choctaws during the Trail of Tears. Wheelock was open only to girls, aged ten to sixteen years, and they were taught in English, given English names, and forbidden to speak *Chahta*. Curriculum included sewing, making clothing, and doing household chores. They also learned reading, writing, and spelling, and special courses included arithmetic, music, and geography. In 1932, Wheelock became a U.S. Indian school; it closed permanently in 1955. Today it is listed as a National Historic Landmark, with an onsite museum and tours.

5.   Published February 25, 1832, Choctaw Chief George W. Harkins' *Letter to the American People* was printed widely in American newspapers in response to Indian Removal out west.

6.   Choctaws have played *Ishtaboli*, which translates into "little brother of war," for centuries. One of the oldest organized sports, it is an integral part of Choctaw culture and is rough, aggressive, and highly competitive. Once played to settle disputes, it kept warriors strong and fit, ready for possible warfare, as it could be dangerous and last for days.

7.   The Choctaw Nation's constitution emphasizes a social and moral responsibility to its citizens, so profits from business endeavors are reinvested into social

services (e.g., healthcare, housing, and transportation) rather than offered as a per capita payment.

8. This is interesting to me, as tourist engagements with Choctaw souvenirs (re) produces the demands for these particular Americana representations of Indianness (and cowboys) and the ways that the tribe participates in a broader colonial racial capitalism that relies on and seeks to perpetuate, reshape, and reapply patterns of (dis)possession and disposability. Remarkably, the dispossession of Indigenous peoples is an unfinished moment in capitalist development that persists and evolves, adapting over time alongside other forms of expropriation and subjugation. As Lisa Cacho (2022) points out, this process involves the "differential devaluation of racialized peoples" and their knowledges, reflecting how these patterns of exploitation remain intertwined with broader systems of inequality and oppression.
9. In 2024, the Choctaw Nation did indeed inaugurate Choctaw Landing, a $238 million luxury resort and casino in Hochatown, Oklahoma, bringing to fruition the plans discussed. Choctaw Landing exemplifies the tribe's strategic shift, featuring one hundred guest rooms (including fifteen suites), a casino with six hundred slot machines and eight table games, multiple dining venues, a fitness center, and an outdoor amphitheater. The resort also integrates Choctaw culture through over six hundred works of art by more than twenty Choctaw artists, including an interactive sculpture by Gene Smith depicting Choctaw social dancers. This development not only serves as an economic engine—creating over four hundred jobs and projecting a $95 million regional impact—but also as a cultural touchstone, aligning with the Nation's efforts to assert a distinct and authentic Choctaw identity in its enterprises.
10. It is interesting to frame this as "counter-authenticity" or "counter-heritage" because then we demand that it co-exist as authentic. We demand recognition of our forms of heritage. Yet, it is still problematic because it is seen as a *counter*-authenticity, a *counter*-heritage.

CHAPTER 5

1. Households may not participate in the FDPIR and Supplemental Nutrition Assistance Program (SNAP) at the same time.
2. Notably, the only items from these two recipes offered in the store are the macaroni pasta and frozen pork chops. The store does not offer taco seasoning, peach preserves, salsa, plastic bags for marinating the pork chops, couscous to serve alongside it, or any of the items required for the pasta salad: Italian dressing, mayonnaise, dill weed, salt, or pepper.
3. UHT (ultra-high temperature) milk has been heated to a higher temperature than regular pasteurized milk, which helps kill more bacteria and significantly extends its shelf life. After heating, it's sealed in aseptic packaging, or sterilized, shelf-stable containers, which keeps it fresh for months without needing refrigeration.

4. The term "paper Indians" is used here to describe people who may be tribally enrolled or officially recognized, but who are seen—within the community—as lacking lived connections to Choctaw culture, land, or practices. In this speaker's account, the distinction between "traditional Choctaws" and "paper Indians" maps onto differences in foodways and embodied experience. It points to deeper questions about authenticity, belonging, and what it means to carry cultural knowledge—especially in relation to food, health, and survival. While the term can carry judgment, it also reflects ongoing struggles over identity, heritage, and the effects of historical and nutritional displacement.

5. To measure participants' perceptions of their current body sizes, I used the Body Image Assessment for Obesity (BIA-O), developed from the original Body Image Assessment (Williamson et al. 1989), which used nine silhouettes of women's figures, ranging from very thin to overweight in body size. The developers expanded the BIA for use with obese persons by creating nine additional silhouettes for men and women, which were constructed to be identical in form to the original figures. BIA-O figures begin at a size larger than the largest BIA figure and show progressively larger body sizes ranging from an overweight body size to a very obese body size. For this study, each silhouette was approximately 6.5 inches in height and was presented to participants on individual, laminated cards the size of a standard sheet of paper (8.5 × 11 inches) (Williamson et al. 2000).

6. Only the first question, "Which silhouette most accurately depicts your current body size?" is validated in the literature. The additional discussions arose because, during most of the interviews, women offered (without prompting) which body size they would like to be, what they thought was healthy and unhealthy, and then joked about Choctaw bodies compared to white bodies. Participants were asked to be honest and to choose only one silhouette. I recorded the number (which is written on the back of the card, so the participant could not use the number as an aid in selecting a body size estimate) for each of the six questions, which is the score for the following domains: 1) Current Body Size; 2) Ideal Body Size; 3) Healthy Body Size; 4) Unhealthy Body Size; 5) Choctaw Body Size; 6) White Body Size.

7. BIA-O scores are as follows: underweight scores range from 1–5; normal weight scores range from 6–9; overweight scores range from 10–13; and obese weight scores range from 14–18 (Williamson et al. 2000).

8. The BMI was calculated for each participant using the National Institutes of Health BMI Calculator, which divides body mass by the square of body height. The BMI range for all participants was 18.3–52, with a mean BMI of 33.9 (± 7.7). Of all participants, 63 percent were categorized as obese, with approximately 41 percent severely or very severely obese. The BMI is widely criticized as an inadequate measure of health because it oversimplifies complex aspects of body composition by relying solely on weight and height. It does not distinguish between muscle, fat, or bone mass, leading to misleading classifications such

as labeling muscular individuals as overweight or obese and failing to account for fat distribution, which is a more accurate predictor of health risks. Furthermore, the BMI does not consider factors like age, sex, or ethnicity, which are critical to understanding an individual's health profile. For instance, studies show that the BMI tends to misclassify health risks for different ethnic groups, including Black, Asian, and Indigenous populations. Consequently, its utility as a one-size-fits-all measure is limited. I used the BMI in this research, however, as a way to make sense of size across the sample population and how Choctaw body sizes are mapped onto biomedical understandings of obesity.

9. The "healthy" BIA-O mean was 5.5 [± 1.8] and the unhealthy mean was 12.6 [± 5.2]).

10. Choctaw families are generally very large and inclusive, with gatherings including extended family members (sometimes driving to Oklahoma from Mississippi for gatherings of all types), in-laws, and in-laws' extended families. This is also described as "the Choctaw way."

CONCLUSION

1. Biostatisticians and health demographers are accustomed to measuring life expectancy changes in increments of months, not years. Even small declines in life expectancy such as one tenth or two-tenths of a year indicate that, on a population level, there are a lot more people prematurely dying than is normal (Rabin 2022). These years lost in life expectancy signal a huge and historic impact on the population.

2. This feature was written by Shelia Kirven and Christian Toews, published July 1, 2021 in print and online (https://www.choctawnation.com/biskinik/health /covid-19-stories-of-loss-and-survival/), accessed 11/15/2022.

3. Juking refers to a kind of embodied trick—a quick, sharp move used to fake out your opponent, most often on the basketball court or in field games like football or stickball. It's not just about speed; it's about rhythm and timing, knowing just when to shift your weight or feint a step to the left so the defender takes the bait while you've already gone to the right. To juke someone is to move with intention and deception, to outmaneuver in real time. Beyond sports, it can also describe a kind of everyday misdirection—a way of getting around something or someone through cleverness and movement, often shaped by necessity, instinct, or survival.

BIBLIOGRAPHY

Adabala, Neeharika, Naren Datha, Joseph Joy, Chinmay Kulkarni, Ajay Manchepalli, Aditya Sankar, and Rebecca Walton. 2010. An Interactive Multimedia Framework for Digital Heritage Narratives. *Proceedings of the 18th ACM International Conference on Multimedia (MM '10)* 1445–1448. Association for Computing Machinery, New York. https://doi.org/10.1145/1873951.1874240.

Adams, Elizabeth J., Laurence Grummer-Strawn, and Gilberto Chavez. 2003. Food Insecurity Is Associated with Increased Risk of Obesity in California Women. *The Journal of Nutrition* 133(4):1070–1074.

Akers, Donna L. 2004. *Living in the Land of Death: The Choctaw Nation, 1830–1860*. Michigan State University Press, East Lansing. https://www.jstor.org/stable/10.14321/j.ctt7zt650.

Alexander, Jeffrey C. 2004. Toward a Theory of Cultural Trauma. In *Cultural Trauma and Collective Identity*, edited by Jeffrey C. Alexander, Ron Eyerman, Bernhard Giesen, Neil J. Smelser, Piotr Sztompka, pp. 1–30. University of California Press, Berkeley.

Anderson, Sarah E., and Robert C. Whitaker. 2009. Prevalence of Obesity Among US Preschool Children in Different Racial and Ethnic Groups. *Archives of Pediatrics & Adolescent Medicine* 163(4):344–348. https://doi.org/10.1001/archpediatrics.2009.18.

Anderson, Sue Ann. 1990. Core Indicators of Nutritional State for Difficult-to-Sample Populations. *The Journal of Nutrition* 120(November):1555–1598. https://doi.org/10.1093/jn/120.suppl_11.1555.

Andrasfay, Theresa, and Noreen Goldman. 2021. Association of the COVID-19 Pandemic with Estimated Life Expectancy by Race/Ethnicity in the United States, 2020. *JAMA Network Open* 4(6):e2114520. https://doi.org/10.1001/jamanetworkopen.2021.14520.

Angelantonio, Emanuele Di, Shilpa N. Bhupathiraju, David Wormser, Pei Gao, Stephen Kaptoge, Amy Berrington de Gonzalez, Benjamin J. Cairns, et al. 2016. Body-Mass Index and All-Cause Mortality: Individual-Participant-Data Meta-Analysis of 239 Prospective Studies in Four Continents. *The Lancet* 388(10046):776–86. https://doi.org/10.1016/S0140-6736(16)30175-1.

Arnold, D. 1988. Famine: Social Crisis and Historical Change. *Famine: Social Crisis and Historical Change*. Basil Blackwell, Oxford, United Kingdom. https://www.cabdirect.org/cabdirect/abstract/19891864721.

Atalay, Sonya. 2006. No Sense of the Struggle: Creating a Context for Survivance at the NMAI. *The American Indian Quarterly* 30(3):597–618. https://doi.org/10.1353/aiq.2006.0016.

Baciu, Alina, Yamrot Negussie, Amy Geller, James N. Weinstein, and National Academies of Sciences, Engineering, and Medicine; Health and Medicine Division; Board on Population Health and Public Health Practice; Committee on Community-Based Solutions to Promote Health Equity in the United States. 2017. *Communities in Action: Pathways to Health Equity*. National Academies Press (US), Washington, D.C. https://www.ncbi.nlm.nih.gov/books/NBK 425854/.

Banner, Stuart. 2005. *How the Indians Lost Their Land: Law and Power on the Frontier*. Harvard University Press, Cambridge, Massachusetts. https://doi.org/10.4159/9780674020535.

Barker, Joanne. 2011. *Native Acts: Law, Recognition, and Cultural Authenticity*. Duke University Press, Durham, North Carolina.

Barnes, Ann Smith. 2011. The Epidemic of Obesity and Diabetes. *Texas Heart Institute Journal* 38(2):142–144.

Barth, Fredrik. 1969. Pathan Identity and Its Maintenance. In *Ethnic Groups and Boundaries: The Social Organization of Culture Difference*, edited by Fredrik Barth, pp. 117–134. Universitets Forlaget, Bergen, Norway.

Beardsworth, Alan, and Teresa Keil. 2002. *Sociology on the Menu: An Invitation to the Study of Food and Society*. Routledge, New York and London.

Beauman, Christopher, Geoffrey Cannon, Ibrahim Elmadfa, Peter Glasauer, Ingrid Hoffmann, Markus Keller, Michael Krawinkel, et al. 2005. The Principles, Definition and Dimensions of the New Nutrition Science. *Public Health Nutrition* 8(6a):695–698. https://doi.org/10.1079/PHN2005820.

Belcourt, Billy-Ray. 2018. Meditations on Reserve Life, Biosociality, and the Taste of Non-Sovereignty. *Settler Colonial Studies* 8(1):1–15. https://doi.org/10.1080/2201 473X.2017.1279830.

Bell, Ricky, Catherine Smith, Leigh Hale, Geoffrey Kira, and Steve Tumilty. 2017. Understanding Obesity in the Context of an Indigenous Population—A Qualitative Study. *Obesity Research & Clinical Practice* 11(5):558–566. https://doi.org/10.1016/j.orcp.2017.04.006.

Bellamy, Leanne, Juan-Pablo Casas, Aroon D Hingorani, and David Williams. 2009. Type 2 Diabetes Mellitus after Gestational Diabetes: A Systematic Review and

Meta-Analysis. *The Lancet* 373(9677):1773–1779. https://doi.org/10.1016/S0140 -6736(09)60731-5.

Bendix, Regina. 2002. Capitalizing on Memories Past, Present, and Future: Observations on the Intertwining of Tourism and Narration. *Anthropological Theory* 2(4):469–487. https://doi.org/10.1177/14634990260620567.

Berger, Leslie. 1988. The Long-Term Psychological Consequences of the Holocaust on the Survivors and Their Offspring. In *The Psychological Perspectives of the Holocaust and of Its Aftermath*, edited by Randolph Braham, pp. 175–221. Holocaust Studies Series Vol. 11. Social Science Monographs, Ann Arbor, Michigan. http://psycnet.apa.org/psycinfo/1988-98245-010.

Berlant, Lauren. 2007. Slow Death (Sovereignty, Obesity, Lateral Agency). *Critical Inquiry* 33(4):754–80. https://doi.org/10.1086/521568.

Bisogni, Carole A., Margaret Connors, Carol M. Devine, and Jeffery Sobal. 2002. Who We Are and How We Eat: A Qualitative Study of Identities in Food Choice. *Journal of Nutrition Education and Behavior* 34(3):128–39. https://doi.org/10 .1016/S1499-4046(06)60082-1.

Blackstock, Cindy, Dawn Bruyere, Elizabeth Moreau, and Canadian Paediatric Society. 2006. *Many Hands, One Dream: Principles for a New Perspective on the Health of First Nations, Inuit, and Métis Children and Youth*. Canadian Paediatric Society, Ottawa.

Bloomgarden, Zachary T. 2004. Type 2 Diabetes in the Young: The Evolving Epidemic. *Diabetes Care* 27(4):998–1010. https://doi.org/10.2337/diacare.27.4.998.

Bochner, Arthur, and Nicholas A. Riggs. 2014. Practicing Narrative Inquiry. In *The Oxford Handbook of Qualitative Research*, edited by Patricia Leavy, pp. 195–222.

Bodirsky, Monica, and Jon Johnson. 2008. Decolonizing Diet: Healing by Reclaiming Traditional Indigenous Foodways. *Cuizine: The Journal of Canadian Food CulturesCuizine:/Revue Des Cultures Culinaires Au Canada* 1(1). http://www.erudit .org/revue/cuizine/2008/v1/n1/019373ar.html.

Bombay, Amy, Kimberly Matheson, and Hymie Anisman. 2014. The Intergenerational Effects of Indian Residential Schools: Implications for the Concept of Historical Trauma. *Transcultural Psychiatry* 51(3):320–38. https://doi.org/10.1177 /1363461513503380.

Bourdieu, Pierre. 1998. *Acts of Resistance*. New Press, New York. http://digamo.free .fr/bourdieu98.pdf.

Bourdieu, Pierre. 2001. *Masculine Domination*. Stanford University Press, Redwood City, California.

Bourgois, Philippe I., and Jeff Schonberg. 2009. *Righteous Dopefiend*. California Series in Public Anthropology Vol. 21. University of California Press, Oakland.

Brave Heart, Maria Yellow Horse. 1999. Gender Differences in the Historical Trauma Response Among the Lakota. *Journal of Health & Social Policy* 10(4):1–20.

Brave Heart, Maria Yellow Horse. 1999. Oyate Ptayela: Rebuilding the Lakota Nation through Addressing Historical Trauma among Lakota Parents. *Journal of Human Behavior in the Social Environment* 2(1/2):109–26.

Brave Heart, Maria Yellow Horse. 2003. The Historical Trauma Response among Natives and Its Relationship with Substance Abuse: A Lakota Illustration. *Journal of Psychoactive Drugs* 35(1):7–13.

Brave Heart, Maria Yellow Horse. 2004. The Historical Trauma Response among Natives and Its Relationship to Substance Abuse: A Lakota Illustration. In *Healing and Mental Health for Native Americans: Speaking in Red.*, edited by Ethan Nebelkopf and Mary Phillips, pp. 7–18. AltaMira Press, Walnut Creek, California.

Brave Heart, Maria Yellow Horse, Josephine Chase, Jennifer Elkins, and Deborah B. Altschul. 2011. Historical Trauma among Indigenous Peoples of the Americas: Concepts, Research, and Clinical Considerations. *Journal of Psychoactive Drugs* 43(4):282–90.

Brave Heart, Maria Yellow Horse, and Lemyra M. DeBruyn. 1998. The American Indian Holocaust: Healing Historical Unresolved Grief. *American Indian and Alaska Native Mental Health Research* 8(2):60–82.

Brave Heart, Maria Yellow Horse, and Tina Deschenie. 2006. Resource Guide: Historical Trauma and Post-Colonial Stress in American Indian Populations. *Tribal College Journal of American Indian Higher Education* 17(3).

Brave Heart-Jordan, Maria Yellow Horse. 1995. The Return to the Sacred Path: Healing from Historical Trauma and Historical Unresolved Grief among the Lakota. PhD dissertation, School for Social Work, Smith College, Northampton, Massachusetts.

Braveheart-Jordan, Maria, and Lemyra DeBruyn. 1995. So She May Walk in Balance: Integrating the Impact of Historical Trauma in the Treatment of Native American Indian Women. In *Racism in the Lives of Women: Testimony, Theory, and Guides to Antiracist Practice.*, edited by Jeanne Adleman and Gloria M. Enguídanos, 345–68. Haworth Innovations in Feminist Studies. Harrington Park Press/Haworth Press, New York.

Brewis, Alexandra A. 2011. *Obesity: Cultural and Biocultural Perspectives*. Rutgers University Press, New Brunswick, New Jersey.

Briggs, Rachel V. 2015. The Hominy Foodway of the Historic Native Eastern Woodlands. *Native South* 8(1):112–46. https://doi.org/10.1353/nso.2015.0004.

Brockett, Charles D. (editor). 1991. *Land, Power, and Poverty: Agrarian Transformation and Political Conflict in Central America*. Routledge, New York and London.

Brones, Anna. 2018. Food Apartheid: The Root of the Problem with America's Groceries. *The Guardian*, May 15, 2018. http://www.theguardian.com/society/2018/may/15/food-apartheid-food-deserts-racism-inequality-america-karen-washington-interview.

Broussard Brenda A., Jonathan R. Sugarman, Karen Bachman-Carter, Karmen Booth, Larry Stephenson, Karen Strauss, and Dorothy Gohdes. 1995. Toward Comprehensive Obesity Prevention Programs in Native American Communities. *Obesity Research* 3(S2): 289s–297s. https://doi.org/10.1002/j.1550-8528.1995.tb00476.x.

Brown, Linda Keller, and Kay Mussell. 1984. *Ethnic and Regional Foodways in the United States: The Performance of Group Identity*. University of Tennessee Press, Knoxville, Tennessee.

Bucholtz, Mary, and Kira Hall. 2004. Theorizing Identity in Language and Sexuality Research. *Language in Society* 33(4):469–515.

Bucholtz, Mary, and Kira Hall. 2005. Language and Identity. In *A Companion to Linguistic Anthropology*, edited by Alessandro Duranti, pp. 369–94. Wiley-Blackwell, Hoboken, New Jersey. https://doi.org/10.1002/9780470996522.ch16.

Burkitt, Ian. 1991. *Social Selves: Theories of the Social Formation of Personality*. Sage, London.

Burt, Larry W. 1986. Roots of the Native American Urban Experience: Relocation Policy in the 1950s. *American Indian Quarterly* 10(2):85–99. https://doi.org/10.2307/1183982.

Byrd, Jodi A. 2011. *The Transit of Empire: Indigenous Critiques of Colonialism*. University of Minnesota Press, Minneapolis.

Cacho, Lisa Marie. 2012. *Social Death: Racialized Rightlessness and the Criminalization of the Unprotected*. New York University Press, New York.

Calabrese, Matthew. 2024. Congressional Trust Responsibility and Tribal Health Care. *University of Illinois Law Review Online*, 12.

Calhoun, Lawrence G., and Richard G. Tedeschi. 2014. *Handbook of Posttraumatic Growth: Research and Practice*. Routledge, New York and London.

Candib, Lucy M. 2007. Obesity and Diabetes in Vulnerable Populations: Reflection on Proximal and Distal Causes. *The Annals of Family Medicine* 5(6):547–56. https://doi.org/10.1370/afm.754.

Carson, James Taylor. 2008. "The Obituary of Nations": Ethnic Cleansing, Memory, and the Origins of the Old South. *Southern Cultures* 14(4):6–31.

Cattelino, Jessica R. 2010. The Double Bind of American Indian Need-Based Sovereignty. *Cultural Anthropology* 25(2):235–62.

Centers for Disease Control. 2023. Adult Obesity Prevalence Maps. https://www.cdc.gov/obesity/data-and-statistics/adult-obesity-prevalence-maps.html.

Che, J., and J. Chen. 2001. Food Insecurity in Canadian Households. *Health Reports* 12(4):11–22.

Cherokee Nation v. Georgia. 1831, 30 U.S. 1.

Chino, Michelle, and Lemyra DeBruyn. 2006. Building True Capacity: Indigenous Models for Indigenous Communities. *American Journal of Public Health* 96(4):596.

Choctaw Nation Economic Development Partnership. 2021. *Economic Development Partnership Annual Reports*. 2021. https://www.growchoctaw.com/doingbusiness/annual-reports/.

Choctaw Nation Health Services Authority. 2016. *Choctaw Nation Health*. Choctaw Nation of Oklahoma. https://www.choctawnation.com/about/health/.

Choctaw Nation of Oklahoma. 2016. *Choctaw Nation of Oklahoma: Economic and Demographic Data*. https://www.odot.org/ok-gov-docs/PROGRAMS-AND-PROJECTS/Grants/FASTLANE-US69/REPORTS-TECH-INFO/Tribal%20Data.pdf.

Choctaw Nation of Oklahoma. 2025. Promoting Active Communities Everywhere (PACE). https://www.choctawnation.com/services/pace/.

Chronis, Athinodoros. 2012. Tourists as Story-Builders: Narrative Construction at a Heritage Museum. *Journal of Travel & Tourism Marketing* 29(5):444–459. https://doi.org/10.1080/10548408.2012.691395.

Cohen, Anthony Paul. 1986. *Symbolising Boundaries: Identity and Diversity in British Cultures.* Anthropological Studies of Britain Vol. 2. Manchester University Press, United Kingdom.

Cohen, Felix S. 1982. *Handbook of Federal Indian Law: With Reference Tables and Index.* Lexis Law Publications, New York.

Cornell, Stephen Ellicott. 1988. *The Return of the Native: American Indian Political Resurgence.* Oxford University Press on Demand, Oxford, United Kingdom.

Cornwell, Jocelyn. 1984. *Hard-Earned Lives: Accounts of Health and Illness from East London.* Routledge, New York and London.

Coulthard, Glen. 2014. *Red Skin, White Masks: Rejecting the Colonial Politics of Recognition.* University of Minnesota, Minneapolis.

Counihan, Carole. 1999. *The Anthropology of Food and Body: Gender, Meaning, and Power.* Routledge, New York and London.

Counihan, Carole. 2002. Food as Women's Voice in the San Luis Valley of Colorado. In *Food in the USA: A Reader,* edited by Carole Counihan, pp. 295–304. Routledge, New York and London.

Counihan, Carole, and Penny Van Esterik. 2012. *Food and Culture: A Reader.* Routledge, New York and London.

Coyhis, Don, and Richard Simonelli. 2008. The Native American Healing Experience. *Substance Use & Misuse* 43(12/13):1927–1949.

Crawford, Allison. 2014. 'The Trauma Experienced by Generations Past Having an Effect in Their Descendants': Narrative and Historical Trauma among Inuit in Nunavut, Canada. *Transcultural Psychiatry* 51(3):339–369. https://doi.org/10.1177/1363461512467161.

Cummins, Steven, Ellen Flint, and Stephen A. Matthews. 2014. New Neighborhood Grocery Store Increased Awareness of Food Access but Did Not Alter Dietary Habits or Obesity. *Health Affairs* 33(2):283–291. https://doi.org/10.1377/hlthaff.2013.0512.

Damm, Peter. 2018. Future Risk of Diabetes in Mother and Child after Gestational Diabetes Mellitus. *International Journal of Gynecology & Obstetrics* 104(Supplement):S25–26. https://doi.org/10.1016/j.ijgo.2008.11.025.

Debo, Angie. 1967. *The Rise and Fall of the Choctaw Republic.* The Civilization of the American Indian Vol. 6. University of Oklahoma Press, Norman.

Debo, Angie. 1972. *And Still the Waters Run: The Betrayal of the Five Civilized Tribes.* Princeton Paperbacks Vol. 287. Princeton University Press, New Jersey.

Delgado Bernal, Dolores, Rebeca Burciaga, and Judith Flores Carmona. 2012. Chicana/Latina Testimonios: Mapping the Methodological, Pedagogical, and Political. *Equity & Excellence in Education* 45(3):363–372. https://doi.org/10.1080/10665684.2012.698149.

Dennison, Jean. 2012. *Colonial Entanglement: Constituting a Twenty-First Century Osage Nation.* University of North Carolina Press, Chapel Hill.

Department of Justice. 1995. Office of the Attorney General | Attorney General June 1, 1995, Memorandum on Indian Sovereignty. https://www.justice.gov/archives/ag /attorney-general-june-1-1995-memorandum-indian-sovereignty.

DeRosier, A. H. 1970. *The Removal of the Choctaw Indians*. University of Tennessee Press, Knoxville.

Dicks, Bella. 2000. *Heritage, Place and Community*. University of Wales Press, Cardiff, United Kingdom.

Dillinger, Teresa. 1999. Feast or Famine? Supplemental Food Programs and Their Impacts on Two American Indian Communities in California. *International Journal of Food Sciences and Nutrition* 50(3):173–187.

Douglas, Mary. 1966. *Purity and Danger: An Analysis of Concepts of Pollution and Taboo*. Routledge, New York and London.

Dressler, William W. 1993. Health in the African American Community: Accounting for Health Inequalities. *Medical Anthropology Quarterly* 7(4):325–345.

Dressler, William W., Kathryn S. Oths, and Clarence C. Gravlee. 2005. Race and Ethnicity in Public Health Research: Models to Explain Health Disparities. *Annual Review of Anthropology* 34(1):231–252. https://doi.org/10.1146/annurev.anthro .34.081804.120505.

Dubowitz, Tamara, Madhumita Ghosh-Dastidar, Deborah A. Cohen, Robin Beckman, Elizabeth D. Steiner, Gerald P. Hunter, Karen R. Flórez, Christina Huang, Christine A. Vaughan, and Jennifer C. Sloan. 2015. Diet and Perceptions Change with Supermarket Introduction in a Food Desert, but Not Because of Supermarket Use. *Health Affairs* 34(11):1858–1868.

Duran, Eduardo, and Bonnie Duran. 1995. *Native American Postcolonial Psychology*. State University of New York Press, Albany.

Dutt, Priyanka, Anastasya Fateyeva, Michelle Gabereau, and Marc Higgins. 2022. Redrawing Relationalities at the Anthropocene(s): Disrupting and Dismantling the Colonial Logics of Shared Identity Through Thinking with Kim Tallbear. In *Reimagining Science Education in the Anthropocene* Vol. 1, edited by Maria F. G. Wallace, Jesse Bazzul, Marc Higgins, and Sara Tolbert, pp. 109–120.

Edelheim, Johan R. 2015. *Tourist Attractions: From Object to Narrative*. Channel View Publications, Bristol, United Kingdom.

Elias, Brenda, Javier Mignone, Madelyn Hall, Say P. Hong, Lyna Hart, and Jitender Sareen. 2012. Trauma and Suicide Behaviour Histories among a Canadian Indigenous Population: An Empirical Exploration of the Potential Role of Canada's Residential School System. *Social Science & Medicine* 74(10):1560–1569.

Emmerich, Samuel, Cheryl Fryar, Bryan Stierman, and Cynthia Ogden. 2024. Obesity and Severe Obesity Prevalence in Adults: United States, August 2021–August 2023. National Center for Health Statistics (U.S.). https://doi.org/10.15620/cdc /159281.

Evans-Campbell, T. 2008. Historical Trauma in American Indian/Native Alaska Communities: A Multilevel Framework for Exploring Impacts on Individuals, Families, and Communities. *Journal of Interpersonal Violence* 23(3):316–338.

Eyerman, Ron. 2001. *Cultural Trauma: Slavery and the Formation of African American Identity*. Cambridge University Press, United Kingdom.

Faiman-Silva, Sandra. 1993. Decolonizing the Choctaw Nation: Choctaw Political Economy in the Twentieth Century. *American Indian Culture and Research Journal* 17(2):43–73.

Faiman-Silva, Sandra. 2000. *Choctaws at the Crossroads: The Political Economy of Class and Culture in the Oklahoma Timber Region*. University of Nebraska Press, Lincoln.

Farmer, P. 1999. Pathologies of Power: Rethinking Health and Human Rights. *American Journal of Public Health* 89(10):1486–1496. https://doi.org/10.2105/AJPH.89.10.1486.

Farmer, Paul. 1996. On Suffering and Structural Violence: A View from Below. *Daedalus* 125(1):261–283.

Farmer, Paul. 2004. An Anthropology of Structural Violence. *Current Anthropology* 45(3):305–325. https://doi.org/10.1086/382250.

Farmer, Paul. 2006. *AIDS and Accusation: Haiti and the Geography of Blame*. University of California Press, Berkeley.

Fee, Margery. 2006. Racializing Narratives: Obesity, Diabetes and the 'Aboriginal' Thrifty Genotype. *Social Science & Medicine* 62(12):2988–2997.

Ferreira, Mariana K. Leal, and Gretchen Chesley Lang, eds. 2006. *Indigenous Peoples and Diabetes: Community Empowerment and Wellness*. Medical Anthropology Series. Carolina Academic Press, Durham, North Carolina.

Flegal, Katherine M., and Kamyar Kalantar-Zadeh. 2013. Overweight, Mortality and Survival. *Obesity* 21(9):1744–1745.

Foreman, Grant. 1932. *Indian Removal: The Emigration of the Five Civilized Tribes of Indians*. University of Oklahoma Press, Norman.

Frideres, James. 2008. Aboriginal Identity in the Canadian Context. *The Canadian Journal of Native Studies* 28(2):313–342.

Galtung, Johan. 1969. Violence, Peace, and Peace Research. *Journal of Peace Research* 6(3):167–191. https://doi.org/10.1177/002234336900600301.

Ganz, Elissa. 2002. Intergenerational Transmission of Trauma: Grandchildren of Holocaust Survivors. PhD dissertation, The Gordon F. Derner Institute of Advanced Psychological Studies, Adelphi University, Garden City, New York.

Garine, Igor and Pollock De. 2013. *Social Aspects of Obesity*. Routledge, New York and London.

Garrett, Michael Tlanusta, and Eugene F. Pichette. 2000. Red as an Apple: Native American Acculturation and Counseling with or without Reservation. *Journal of Counseling & Development* 78(1):3–13. https://doi.org/10.1002/j.1556-6676.2000.tb02554.x.

Gibson, Diane. 2003. Food Stamp Program Participation Is Positively Related to Obesity in Low Income Women. *The Journal of Nutrition* 133(7):2225–2231.

Gittelsohn, Joel, Stewart B. Harris, Krista L. Burris, Louisa Kakegamic, Laura T. Landman, Anjali Sharma, Thomas M. S. Wolever, Alexander Logan, Annette Barnie, and Bernard Zinman. 1996. Use of Ethnographic Methods for Applied Research on Diabetes among the Ojibway-Cree in Northern Ontario. *Health Education & Behavior* 23(3):365–382.

Gone, Joseph P. 2013. Redressing First Nations Historical Trauma: Theorizing Mechanisms for Indigenous Culture as Mental Health Treatment. *Transcultural Psychiatry* 50(5):683–706. https://doi.org/10.1177/1363461513487669.

Gone, Joseph P. 2014. Reconsidering American Indian Historical Trauma: Lessons from an Early Gros Ventre War Narrative. *Transcultural Psychiatry* 51(3):387–406. https://doi.org/10.1177/1363461513489722.

Gone, Joseph P., and Laurence J. Kirmayer. 2010. On the Wisdom of Considering Culture and Context in Psychopathology. In *Contemporary Directions in Psychopathology: Scientific Foundations of the DSM-V and ICD-11*, edited by Theodore Millon, Robert F. Krueger, and Erik Simonsen, pp. 72–96. The Guilford Press, New York.

Gone, Joseph P., and Joseph E. Trimble. 2012. American Indian and Alaska Native Mental Health: Diverse Perspectives on Enduring Disparities. *Annual Review of Clinical Psychology* 8(1):131–160. https://doi.org/10.1146/annurev-clinpsy-032511 -143127.

Goodman, Alan H., and Thomas L. Leatherman. 1998. Traversing the Chasm between Biology and Culture: An Introduction. In *Building a New Biocultural Synthesis: Political-Economic Perspectives on Human Biology*, edited by Alan H. Goodman and Thomas L. Leatherman, pp. 3-41. University of Michigan Press, Ann Arbor.

Graesch, Anthony, Julienne Bernard, and Anna Noah. 2010. A Cross-Cultural Study of Colonialism and Indigenous Foodways in Western North America. In *Across a Great Divide: Continuity and Change in Native North American Societies, 1400–1900*, edited by Laura L. Scheiber and Mark D. Mitchell, pp. 212–238. University of Arizona Press, Tucson.

Graham, Brian, Gregory John Ashworth, and John E. Tunbridge. 2000. *A Geography of Heritage: Power, Culture, and Economy*. Oxford University Press, Arnold. http://www.bcin.ca/Interface/openbcin.cgi?submit=submit&Chinkey=205479.

Graham, Brian J., and Peter Howard. 2008. *The Ashgate Research Companion to Heritage and Identity*. Ashgate Publishing, Farnham, United Kingdom.

Gravlee, Clarence C., William W. Dressler, and H. Russell Bernard. 2005. Skin Color, Social Classification, and Blood Pressure in Southeastern Puerto Rico. *American Journal of Public Health* 95(12):2191–2197. https://doi.org/10.2105/AJPH.2005 .065615.

Greenberg, James A. 2013. Obesity and Early Mortality in the United States. *Obesity* 21(2):405–412. https://doi.org/10.1002/oby.20023.

Greenhalgh, Susan, and Megan A. Carney. 2014. Bad Biocitizens? Latinos and the US 'Obesity Epidemic.' *Human Organization* 73(3):267–276. https://doi.org/10 .17730/humo.73.3.w53hh1t413038240.

Hake, M., A. Dewey, E. Engelhard, and S. Dawes. 2024. Map the Meal Gap 2024: A Report on County and Congressional District Food Insecurity and County

Food Cost in the United States in 2022. Feeding America, Chicago. https://www .feedingamerica.org/research/map-the-meal-gap/overall-executive-summary.

Hall, James. 2015. The Promise Zone Initiative and Native American Economic Development: Only the First Step Forward toward the Promise of a Brighter Future. *American Indian Law Review* 40:249.

Halpern, Peggy. 2007. Obesity and American Indians/Alaska Natives. United States Department of Health and Human Services, Washington, D.C. http://aspe.hhs .gov/hsp/07/AI-AN-obesity/.

Hammond, Ross A., and Ruth Levine. 2010. The Economic Impact of Obesity in the United States. *Diabetes, Metabolic Syndrome and Obesity: Targets and Therapy* 3(August):285–295. https://doi.org/10.2147/DMSOTT.S7384.

Hanson, Arlen M. 2021. Troubled Voices: Choctaws in Mass Deportation and Ethnic Cleansing. PhD dissertation, Graduate School, University of North Carolina at Greensboro. https://search.proquest.com/openview/604621d49dcaa24015c18 2c7e892e2a0/1?pq-origsite=gscholar&cbl=18750&diss=y.

Harris, Ben, and Aurite Werman. 2014. The High Cost of Obesity on Government Budgets. Brookings Institution, December 12, 2014. https://www.brookings.edu /articles/obesity-costs-evident-at-the-state-level/.

Harrison, Rodney. 2009. Excavating Second Life: Cyber-Archaeologies, Heritage and Virtual Communities. *Journal of Material Culture* 14(1):75–106. https://doi.org /10.1177/1359183508100009.

Hartmann, William E., and Joseph P. Gone. 2014. American Indian Historical Trauma: Community Perspectives from Two Great Plains Medicine Men. *American Journal of Community Psychology* 54(3–4), 274–288.

Harvey, David C. 2001. Heritage Pasts and Heritage Presents: Temporality, Meaning and the Scope of Heritage Studies. *International Journal of Heritage Studies* 7(4):319–338.

Hauck-Lawson, Annie S. 1998. When Food Is the Voice: A Case Study of a Polish-American Woman. *Journal for the Study of Food and Society* 2(1):21–28. https:// doi.org/10.2752/152897998786690592.

Healy, Jack, and Adam Liptak. 2020. Landmark Supreme Court Ruling Affirms Native American Rights in Oklahoma. *The New York Times*, July 9, 2020, sec. U.S. https://www.nytimes.com/2020/07/09/us/supreme-court-oklahoma-mcgirt -creek-nation.html.

Heart, Brave, and Lemyra M. DeBruyn. 1998. The American Indian Holocaust: Healing Historical Unresolved Grief. *American Indian and Alaska Native Mental Health Research* 8(2):56–78.

Heil, Daniela. 2008. "4 EMBODIED SELVES AND SOCIAL SELVES: Aboriginal Well-Being in Rural New South Wales, Australia." In *Pursuits of Happiness: Well-Being in Anthropological Perspective*, edited by Gordon Mathews and Carolina Izquierdo, pp. 88–108. Berghahn Books, New York and Oxford. https://doi.org /10.1515/9781845458775-008.

Herrera, Allison. 2021. 'We're Not Going Anywhere': Choctaw Freedmen Cite History, Ties to Tribal Nation in Fight for Citizenship. KOSU, Oklahoma City, September 22, 2021. https://www.kosu.org/local-news/2021-09-22/were-not-going-anywhere -choctaw-freedmen-cite-history-ties-to-tribal-nation-in-fight-for-citizenship.

Herring, Sharon J., and Emily Oken. 2011. Obesity and Diabetes in Mothers and Their Children: Can We Stop the Intergenerational Cycle? *Current Diabetes Reports* 11(1):20–27. https://doi.org/10.1007/s11892-010-0156-9.

Hill, Andrew J., and Inge Lissau. 2006. Psychosocial Factors. In *Child and Adolescent Obesity: Causes and Consequences, Prevention and Management*, edited by Walter Burniat, Tim Cole, Inge Lissau, and Elizabeth Poskitt, pp. 109–127. Cambridge University Press, Cambridge, United Kingdom.

Hurt, R. Douglas. 1987. *Indian Agriculture in America: Prehistory to the Present*. University Press of Kansas, Lawrence. http://agris.fao.org/agris-search/search.do ?recordID=US8919912.

Hutto, Stacy. 2017. Changes on the Horizon for Food Distribution Program. *Biskinik*, June. https://www.choctawnation.com/wp-content/uploads/2022/06/jun -2017-biskinik.pdf.

Intertribal Agriculture Council. 2018. Intertribal Agriculture Council (blog). May 21. http://www.indianag.org/news.

Iti Fabvssa. 2010. Choctaw Place Names in 'Oklahumma'. *Biskinik*, September 2010.

Jaimes, M. Annette. 1992. Federal Indian Identification Policy: A Usurpation of Indigenous Sovereignty in North American. *Native Americans and Public Policy*, 113–135.

Janoff-Bulman, Ronnie, and Sana Sheikh. 2006. From National Trauma to Moralizing Nation. *Basic and Applied Social Psychology* 28(4):325–32. https://doi.org/10 .1207/s15324834basp2804_5.

Jernigan, Kasey. 2013. Commod Bod: The Embodiment of Commodity Food Programs on American Indian Reservations. Paper presented at the 73rd Annual Meeting for the Society for Applied Anthropology: Natural Resource Distribution and Development in the 21st Century, Denver, Colorado, March 21.

Jernigan, Kasey Aliene. 2018. Embodied Heritage: Obesity, Cultural Identity, and Food Distribution Programs in the Choctaw Nation of Oklahoma. PhD dissertation, Graduate School, University of Massachusetts, Amherst. https://hdl.handle .net/20.500.14394/17565.

Joe, Jennie Rose, and Robert S. Young. 1994. *Diabetes as a Disease of Civilization: The Impact of Culture Change on Indigenous Peoples*. Mouton de Gruyter, Berlin.

Jones, David S. 2006. The Persistence of American Indian Health Disparities. *American Journal of Public Health* 96(12):2122–2134. https://doi.org/10.2105/AJPH .2004.054262.

Joseph, Stephen, and P. Alex Linley. 2005. Positive Adjustment to Threatening Events: An Organismic Valuing Theory of Growth Through Adversity. *Review of General Psychology* 9(3):262–280. https://doi.org/10.1037/1089-2680.9.3.262.

Josselson, Ruthellen. 2011. Narrative Research: Constructing, Deconstructing, and Reconstructing Story. In *Five Ways of Doing Qualitative Analysis: Phenomenological Psychology, Grounded Theory, Discourse Analysis, Narrative Research, and Intuitive Inquiry*, edited by Frederick J. Wertz, Kathy Charmaz, Linda M. McMullen, Ruthellen Josselson, Rosemarie Anderson, and Emalinda McSpadden, pp. 224–242. Guildford Press, New York.

Kidron, Carol A. 2012. Alterity and the Particular Limits of Universalism: Comparing Jewish-Israeli Holocaust and Canadian-Cambodian Genocide Legacies. *Current Anthropology* 53(6):723–754. https://doi.org/10.1086/668449.

Kirmayer, Laurence J., Joseph P. Gone, and Joshua Moses. 2014. "Rethinking Historical Trauma." *Transcultural Psychiatry* 51 (3): 299–319. https://doi.org/10.1177/1363461514536358.

Kleinman, Arthur. 1997. "Everything That Really Matters": Social Suffering, Subjectivity, and the Remaking of Human Experience in a Disordering World. *Harvard Theological Review* 90(3):315–336.

Kleinman, Arthur. 2001. The Violences of Everyday Life: The Multiple Forms and Dynamics of Social Violence. In *Violence and Subjectivity*, edited by Veena Das, Arthur Kleinman, Mamphela Ramphele, and Pamela Reynolds, pp. 226–41. University of California Press, Oakland. https://doi.org/10.1525/9780520921825-011.

Kleinman, Arthur, Leon Eisenberg, and Byron Good. 1978. Culture, Illness, and Care-Clinical Lessons from Anthropologic and Cross-Cultural Research. *Annals of Internal Medicine* 88(2):251–258. https://doi.org/10.7326/0003-4819-88-2-251.

Kompaniyets, Lyudmyla. 2021. Body Mass Index and Risk for COVID-19–Related Hospitalization, Intensive Care Unit Admission, Invasive Mechanical Ventilation, and Death: United States, March–December 2020. *MMWR. Morbidity and Mortality Weekly Report* 70. https://www.cdc.gov/mmwr/volumes/70/wr/mm7010e4.htm?s%5C_cid=mm7010e4%5C_w.

Krauthamer, Barbara. 2013. *Black Slaves, Indian Masters: Slavery, Emancipation, and Citizenship in the Native American South*. University of North Carolina Press, Chapel Hill.

Krieger, Nancy. 2001. Theories for Social Epidemiology in the 21st Century: An Ecosocial Perspective. *International Journal of Epidemiology* 30(4):668–677.

Krieger, Nancy. 2005. Embodiment: A Conceptual Glossary for Epidemiology. *Journal of Epidemiology and Community Health* 59(5):350–355. https://doi.org/10.1136/jech.2004.024562.

Lambert, Valerie. 2007. *Choctaw Nation: A Story of American Indian Resurgence*. University of Nebraska Press, Lincoln.

Lang, Gretchen Chesley. 2006. 'In Their Tellings': Dakota Narratives about History and the Body. In *Indigenous Peoples and Diabetes: Community Empowerment and Wellness*, edited by Mariana Leal Ferreira and Gretchen Chesley Lang, pp. 53–71. Carolina Academic Press, Durham, North Carolina.

Laraia, Barbara A., Anna Maria Siega-Riz, Jay S. Kaufman, and Sonya J. Jones. 2004. Proximity of Supermarkets Is Positively Associated with Diet Quality Index for

Pregnancy. *Preventive Medicine* 39(5):869–875. https://doi.org/10.1016/j.ypmed
.2004.03.018.

Lauby-Secretan, Béatrice, Chiara Scoccianti, Dana Loomis, Yann Grosse, Franca Bi-
anchini, Kurt Straif, and International Agency for Research on Cancer Handbook
Working Group. 2016. Body Fatness and Cancer: Viewpoint of the IARC Working
Group. *The New England Journal of Medicine* 375(8):794–798. https://doi.org/10
.1056/NEJMsr1606602.

Leatherman, Thomas. 2005. A Space of Vulnerability in Poverty and Health: Political-
Ecology and Biocultural Analysis. *Ethos* 33(1):46–70. https://doi.org/10.1525/eth
.2005.33.1.046.

Leatherman, Tom, and Alan H. Goodman. 2011. Critical Biocultural Approaches
in Medical Anthropology. In *A Companion to Medical Anthropology*, edited by
Merrill Singer and Pamela I. Erickson, pp. 29–48. Wiley-Blackwell, Hoboken,
New Jersey. https://doi.org/10.1002/9781444395303.ch2.

Leddy, Meaghan A, Michael L Power, and Jay Schulkin. 2008. The Impact of Maternal Obesity on Maternal and Fetal Health. *Reviews in Obstetrics and Gynecology*
1(4):170–178.

Lee, Helen. 2012. The Role of Local Food Availability in Explaining Obesity Risk
among Young School-Aged Children. *Social Science & Medicine* 74(8):1193–1203.
https://doi.org/10.1016/j.socscimed.2011.12.036.

Littlefield Jr, Daniel F. 1978. *The Cherokee Freedmen: From Emancipation to American
Citizenship*. Bloomsbury Publishing, New York.

Lock, Margaret. 2001. The Tempering of Medical Anthropology: Troubling Natural
Categories. *Medical Anthropology Quarterly* 15(4):478–492.

Lock, Margaret M., and Judith Farquhar. 2007. *Beyond the Body Proper: Reading the Anthropology of Material Life*. Duke University Press, Durham, North
Carolina.

Loulanski, Tolina. 2006. Revising the Concept for Cultural Heritage: The Argument for a Functional Approach. *International Journal of Cultural Property*
13(2):207–233.

Lowenthal, David. 1985. *The Past Is a Foreign Country*. Cambridge University Press,
United Kingdom.

Lowenthal, David. 1998. Fabricating Heritage. *History and Memory* 10(1):5–24.

Lowrey, Annie. 2021. The Time Tax. *The Atlantic* (blog), July 27, 2021. https://www
.theatlantic.com/politics/archive/2021/07/how-government-learned-waste-your
-time-tax/619568/.

Mai, Xiao-Mei, Allan B. Becker, Elizabeth A. C. Sellers, Joel J. Liem, and Anita L.
Kozyrskyj. 2007. The Relationship of Breast-Feeding, Overweight, and Asthma
in Preadolescents. *Journal of Allergy and Clinical Immunology* 120(3):551–556.
https://doi.org/10.1016/j.jaci.2007.05.004.

Mailer, Gideon, and Nicola Hale. 2015. Decolonizing the Diet: Synthesizing Native-
American History, Immunology, and Nutritional Science. *Journal of Evolution
and Health* 1(1):1–41. https://doi.org/10.15310/2334-3591.1014.

Mani, Anandi, Sendhil Mullainathan, Eldar Shafir, and Jiaying Zhao. 2013. Poverty Impedes Cognitive Function. *Science* 341(6149):976–980. https://doi.org/10.1126 /science.1238041.

Martin, Katie S., and Ann M. Ferris. 2007. Food Insecurity and Gender Are Risk Factors for Obesity. *Journal of Nutrition Education and Behavior* 39(1):31–36. https://doi.org/10.1016/j.jneb.2006.08.021.

Mascia-Lees, Frances E. 2011. *A Companion to the Anthropology of the Body and Embodiment.* Wiley-Blackwell, Hoboken, New Jersey.

Mauss, Marcel. 1967. *The Gift,* 9th ed. WW Norton & Company, New York and London.

Maxwell, Krista. 2014. Historicizing Historical Trauma Theory: Troubling the Trans-Generational Transmission Paradigm. *Transcultural Psychiatry* 51(3):407–435. https://doi.org/10.1177/1363461514531317.

McBeth, Sally. 1989. Layered Identity Systems in Western Oklahoma Indian Communities. In *Annual Meeting of the American Anthropological Association,* November, Vol. 17.

McDade, Thomas W. 2002. Status Incongruity in Samoan Youth: A Biocultural Analysis of Culture Change, Stress, and Immune Function. *Medical Anthropology Quarterly* 16(2):123–150.

McGirt v. Oklahoma. 2020, 591 U.S. 894.

McKinley, Gerald P. 2012. Narrative Tactics: Windigo Stories and Indigenous Youth Suicide. PhD dissertation, Department of Anthropology, University of Western Ontario, Canada. http://ir.lib.uwo.ca/etd/730/.

McKinnon, Robin A., Jill Reedy, Meredith A. Morrissette, Leslie A. Lytle, and Amy L. Yaroch. 2009. Measures of the Food Environment: A Compilation of the Literature, 1990–2007. *American Journal of Preventive Medicine* 36(4):S124–133. https://doi.org/10.1016/j.amepre.2009.01.012.

McMichael, Anthony J. 1999. Prisoners of the Proximate: Loosening the Constraints on Epidemiology in an Age of Change. *American Journal of Epidemiology* 149(10):887–897.

Meigs, Anna. 1997. Food as a Cultural Construction. In *Food and Culture: A Reader,* edited by Carole Counihan, Penny Van Esterik, and Alice P. Julier, pp. 95–106. Routledge, New York and London.

Meserve, John Bartlett. 1941. Chief Allen Wright. *Chronicles of Oklahoma,* Winter. https://gateway.okhistory.org/ark:/67531/metadc2192214/.

Mihesuah, Devon. 2016. Diabetes in Indian Territory: Revisiting Kelly M. West's Theory of 1940. *American Indian Culture and Research Journal* 40(4):1–21.

Milburn, Michael P. 2004. Indigenous Nutrition: Using Traditional Food Knowledge to Solve Contemporary Health Problems. *The American Indian Quarterly* 28(3):411–434. https://doi.org/10.1353/aiq.2004.0104.

Million, Dian. 2009. Felt Theory: An Indigenous Feminist Approach to Affect and History. *Wicazo Sa Review* 24(2):53–76. https://doi.org/10.1353/wic.0.0043.

Million, Dian. 2013. *Therapeutic Nations: Healing in an Age of Indigenous Human Rights*. University of Arizona Press, Tucson.

Mohatt, Nathaniel Vincent, Azure B. Thompson, Nghi D. Thai, and Jacob Kraemer Tebes. 2014. Historical Trauma as Public Narrative: A Conceptual Review of How History Impacts Present-Day Health. *Social Science & Medicine* 106:128–36.

Moore, John H. 1993. *The Political Economy of North American Indians*. University of Oklahoma Press, Norman.

Morrison, Dane Anthony. 1997. *American Indian Studies: An Interdisciplinary Approach to Contemporary Issues*. Peter Lang Pub, Lausanne, Switzerland.

Nagel, Joane. 1995. American Indian Ethnic Renewal: Politics and the Resurgence of Identity. *American Sociological Review*, 60(6):947–965.

National Archives. Native American Urban Relocation. *Educator Resources*. Electronic document, https://www.archives.gov/education/lessons/indian-relocation.html, accessed August 15, 2016.

National Congress of American Indians. 2018. Indian Country Demographics. Electronic document, http://www.ncai.org/about-tribes/demographics#R1.

National Congress of American Indians. 2020. Tribal Nations & the United States: An Introduction. Electronic Document, https://archive.ncai.org/about-tribes.

National Institute of Diabetes and Digestive and Kidney Diseases. 2023. Health Risks of Overweight & Obesity. Electronic document, https://www.niddk.nih.gov/health-information/weight-management/adult-overweight-obesity/health-risks.

National Institutes of Health. 1998. Clinical Guidelines on the Identification, Evaluation, and Treatment of Overweight and Obesity in Adults: The Evidence Report. NHLBI Obesity Education Initiative Expert Panel on the Identification, Evaluation, and Treatment of Overweight and Obesity in Adults 98–4083. NIH, NHLBI, and NIDDKD. Electronic document, https://www.nhlbi.nih.gov/files/docs/guidelines/ob_gdlns.pdf.

Native American Times. 2011. Choctaw Nation Health Services Announces 'Going Lean.' June 20. https://nativetimes.com/index.php/life/health/5567 choctaw-nation-health-services-announces-going-lean.

Ochs, Elinor, and Lisa Capps. 1996. Narrating the Self. *Annual Review of Anthropology*, 25:19–43. https://doi.org/10.1146/annurev.anthro.25.1.19

O'Connell, Meghan, Dedra S. Buchwald, and Glen E. Duncan. 2011. Food Access and Cost in American Indian Communities in Washington State. *Journal of the American Dietetic Association* 111(9):1375–1379. https://doi.org/10.1016/j.jada.2011.06.002.

Ogden, Cynthia L., Margaret D. Carroll, Brian K. Kit, and Katherine M. Flegal. 2012. Prevalence of Obesity and Trends in Body Mass Index Among US Children and Adolescents, 1999–2010. *JAMA* 307(5):483–490. https://doi.org/10.1001/jama.2012.40.

Oklahoma Employment Security Commission. 2015. Oklahoma Unemployment Rate. Electronic document.

Oklahoma Indian Affairs Commission. 2011. Oklahoma Indian Nations Pocket Pictorial Directory. *Oklahoma Indian Nations Information Handbook*. Publications Clearinghouse of the Oklahoma Department of Libraries, Oklahoma City. www .oiac.ok.gov.

Oklahoma State Department of Health. 2022. State Obesity Plan. Electronic document, https://oklahoma.gov/health/health-education/community-outreach /community-development-services/office-of-state-programs/nutrition-access -and-built-environment/state-obesity-plan.html.

Pareo-Tubbeh, Shirley L., Marvin Shorty, Mark C. Bauer, and Emmanuel Agbolosoo. 2000. The Variety, Affordability, and Availability of Healthful Foods at Convenience Stores and Trading Posts on the Navajo Reservation: Final Report 2000. Native Peoples Technical Assistance Office, University of Arizona, Tucson.

Park, Crystal L., and Amy L. Ai. 2006. Meaning Making and Growth: New Directions for Research on Survivors of Trauma. *Journal of Loss and Trauma* 11(5):389–407. https://doi.org/10.1080/15325020600685295.

Pena, Devon G. 2011. Structural Violence, Historical Trauma, and Public Health: The Environmental Justice Critique of Contemporary Risk Science and Practice. In *Communities, Neighborhoods, and Health: Expanding the Boundaries of Place*, edited by Linda M. Burton, Susan P. Kemp, ManChui Leung, Stephen A. Matthews, and David T. Takeuchi, pp. 203–218. Social Disparities in Health and Health Care. Springer, New York and Heidelberg.

Pilcher, Jeffrey M. 2012. *The Oxford Handbook of Food History*. Oxford University Press, New York.

Plummer, Cheyenne. 2020. *Cherokee Phoenix*. 15 April. Tahlequah, Oklahoma. https://www.cherokeephoenix.org/news/exiled-to-indian-country-choctaw -nation/article_83dbdaf6-ee6d-53d9-968c-7b9c09367aba.html.

Povinelli, Elizabeth A. 2002. *The Cunning of Recognition: Indigenous Alterities and the Making of Australian Multiculturalism*. Duke University Press, Durham, North Carolina.

Prussing, Erica. 2014. Historical Trauma: Politics of a Conceptual Framework. *Transcultural Psychiatry* 51(3):436–458. https://doi.org/10.1177/1363461514531316.

Quesada, James, Laurie Kain Hart, and Philippe Bourgois. 2011. Structural Vulnerability and Health: Latino Migrant Laborers in the United States. *Medical Anthropology* 30(4):339–362. https://doi.org/10.1080/01459740.2011.576725.

Rabin, Roni Caryn. 2022. U.S. Life Expectancy Falls Again in 'Historic' Setback. *The New York Times*, August 31:Health. https://www.nytimes.com/2022/08/31/health /life-expectancy-covid-pandemic.html.

Ramirez, Renya K. 2007. *Native Hubs: Culture, Community, and Belonging in Silicon Valley and Beyond*. Duke University Press, Durham, North Carolina.

Ramshaw, Gregory. 2014. A Canterbury Tale: Imaginative Genealogies and Existential Heritage Tourism at the St. Lawrence Ground. *Journal of Heritage Tourism* 9(3):257–269. https://doi.org/10.1080/1743873X.2014.904319.

Rasmussen, Trond, Lars C. Stene, Sven O. Samuelsen, Ondrej Cinek, Turid Wetlesen, Peter A. Torjesen, and Kjersti S. Rønningen. 2009. Maternal BMI Before Pregnancy, Maternal Weight Gain During Pregnancy, and Risk of Persistent Positivity for Multiple Diabetes-Associated Autoantibodies in Children with the High-Risk HLA Genotype: The MIDIA Study. *Diabetes Care* 32(10):1904–1906. https://doi .org/10.2337/dc09-0663.

Rechtman, Richard. 1997. Transcultural Psychotherapy with Cambodian Refugees in Paris. *Transcultural Psychiatry* 34(3):359–375. https://doi.org/10.1177/136346 159703400305.

Rifkin, Mark. 2017. *Beyond Settler Time: Temporal Sovereignty and Indigenous Self-Determination.* Duke University Press, Durham, North Carolina. https://books .google.com/books?hl=en&lr=&id=y-IZDgAAQBAJ&oi=fnd&pg=PT11&dq= mark+rifkin+beyond+settler+time&ots=dTKJzYswSu&sig=8q9nKYB9y9BfJfP 3eMZ4jxz_fDE.

Roberts, Alaina E. 2021. *I've Been Here All the While: Black Freedom on Native Land.* University of Pennsylvania Press, Philadelphia. https://doi.org/10.9783/978081 2297980.

Roberts, Alaina E. 2023. Black Slaves and Indian Owners: The Continuous Rediscovery of Indian Territory. *The Journal of the Civil War Era* 13(1):87–104.

Roberts, Charles. 1986. The Second Choctaw Removal, 1903. In *After Removal: The Choctaw in Mississippi*, edited by Samuel J. Wells and Roseanna Tubby, pp. 94– 111. University Press of Mississippi, Jackson.

Robertson, Lindsay G. 2005. *Conquest by Law: How the Discovery of America Dispossessed Indigenous Peoples of Their Lands.* Oxford University Press, New York.

Robin, Robert W., Barbara Chester, and David Goldman. 1996. Cumulative Trauma and PTSD in American Indian Communities. In *Ethnocultural Aspects of Posttraumatic Stress Disorder: Issues, Research, and Clinical Applications*, edited by Anthony J. Marsella, Matthew J. Friedman, Ellen T. Gerrity, and Raymond M. Scurfield, pp. 239–253. American Psychological Association, Washington, D.C. http://psycnet.apa.org/psycinfo/1996-97494-009.

Rowland-Klein, Dani, and Rosemary Dunlop. 1998. The Transmission of Trauma across Generations: Identification with Parental Trauma in Children of Holocaust Survivors. *Australian and New Zealand Journal of Psychiatry* 32(3):358–369.

Roy, Bernard. 2005. Diabetes and Identity: Changes in the Food Habits of the Innu. In *Indigenous Peoples and Diabetes: Community Empowerment and Wellness*, edited by Mariana Leal Ferreira and Gretchen Chesley Lang, 167–186. Carolina Academic Press, Durham, North Carolina.

Rubin, Jordan S. 2022. Justices to Hear McGirt-Impact Issue, Not Ditching Precedent (2). *Bloomberg Law*, January 21. https://news.bloomberglaw.com/us-law-week /justices-to-hear-mcgirt-impact-issue-but-wont-ditch-precedent.

Rylko-Bauer, Barbara, and Paul Farmer. 2016. Structural Violence, Poverty, and Social Suffering. In *The Oxford Handbook of the Social Science of Poverty*, edited by David Brady and Linda M. Burton, pp. 47–74. Oxford University Press, New York.

Rylko-Bauer, Barbara, Linda M. Whiteford, and Paul Farmer. 2009. *Global Health in Times of Violence*. School for Advanced Research Press, Santa Fe, New Mexico. http://sarweb.org/media/files/sar_press_global_health_in_times_of_violence _chapter_1.pdf.

Saethre, Eirik. 2013. *Illness Is a Weapon: Indigenous Identity and Enduring Afflictions*. Vanderbilt University Press, Nashville, Tennessee.

Saito, Hiro. 2006. Reiterated Commemoration: Hiroshima as National Trauma*. *Sociological Theory* 24(4):353–376.

Sallis, James F., and Karen Glanz. 2006. The Role of Built Environments in Physical Activity, Eating, and Obesity in Childhood. *The Future of Children* 16(1):89–108.

Saunt, Claudio. 2004. The Paradox of Freedom: Tribal Sovereignty and Emancipation during the Reconstruction of Indian Territory. *The Journal of Southern History* 70(1):63–94.

Saunt, Claudio. 2020. *Unworthy Republic: The Dispossession of Native Americans and the Road to Indian Territory*. WW Norton & Company, New York and London.

Scheder, Jo C. 2006. The Spirit's Cell: Reflections on Diabetes and Political Meaning. In *Indigenous Peoples and Diabetes: Community Empowerment and Wellness*, edited by Mariana Leal Ferreira and Gretchen Chelsey Lang, 335–355. Carolina Academic Press, Durham, North Carolina.

Scheper-Hughes, Nancy. 2004. Dangerous and Endangered Youth: Social Structures and Determinants of Violence. *Annals of the New York Academy of Sciences* 1036(1):13–46. https://doi.org/10.1196/annals.1330.002.

Scheper-Hughes, Nancy, and Philippe I. Bourgois, eds. 2003. *Violence in War and Peace: An Anthology*. Wiley-Blackwell, Hoboken, New Jersey. https://www .academia.edu/download/80844584/9780631223498.pdf.

Schorow, Stephanie. 2010. Candid Chat with Choctaw Chief. *Harvard Gazette*, February 24. https://test.news.harvard.edu/gazette/story/2010/02/candid-chat-with -choctaw-chief/.

Schultz, Katie, Karina L. Walters, Ramona Beltran, Sandy Stroud, and Michelle Johnson-Jennings. 2016. 'I'm Stronger than I Thought': Native Women Reconnecting to Body, Health, and Place. *Health & Place* 40(July):21–28. https://doi .org/10.1016/j.healthplace.2016.05.001.

Sen, Amartya. 1988. Freedom of Choice: Concept and Content. *European Economic Review* 32(2–3):269–294.

Shelton, Brett Lee. 2004. Legal and Historical Roots of Health Care for American Indians and Alaska Natives in the United States. The Henry J. Kaiser Family Foundation. Electronic document, https://www.kff.org/wp-content/uploads/2013/01 /legal-and-historical-roots-of-health-care-for-american-indians-and-alaska -natives-in-the-united-states.pdf.

Simpson, Audra. 2014. *Theorizing Native Studies*. Duke University Press, Durham, North Carolina.

Simpson, Leanne Betasamosake. 2017. *As We Have Always Done: Indigenous Freedom through Radical Resistance*. University of Minnesota Press, Minneapolis.

Singer, Merrill, and Pamela I. Erickson, eds. 2011. *A Companion to Medical Anthropology*, 1st ed. Wiley-Blackwell, Hoboken, New Jersey. https://doi.org/10.1002/9781444395303.

Singer, Merrill, and G. Derrick Hodge. 2010. *The War Machine and Global Health: A Critical Medical Anthropological Examination of the Human Costs of Armed Conflict and the International Violence Industry*. Rowman & Littlefield, Lanham, Maryland.

Smith, George Davey. 2003. *Health Inequalities: Lifecourse Approaches*. The Policy Press, Bristol, United Kingdom.

Smith, Laurajane. 2006. *Uses of Heritage*. Routledge, London and New York. https://doi.org/10.4324/9780203602263.

Smith, Laurajane, Anna Morgan, and Anita van der Meer. 2003. Community-Driven Research in Cultural Heritage Management: The Waanyi Women's History Project. *International Journal of Heritage Studies* 9(1):65–80.

Smith, Marvin T. 1992. *Archaeology of Aboriginal Culture Change in the Interior Southeast : Depopulation during the Early Historic Period*, Ripley P. Bullen Series, Florida Museum of Natural History. University Press of Florida, Gainesville. http://archive.org/details/archaeologyofabo0000smit.

Snipp, C. Matthew. 1992. Sociological Perspectives on American Indians. *Annual Review of Sociology* 18(1):351–371. https://doi.org/10.1146/annurev.so.18.080192.002031.

Snyder, Christina. 2017. *Great Crossings: Indians, Settlers, and Slaves in the Age of Jackson*. Oxford University Press, United Kingdom.

Sobal, Jeffery, Carole A. Bisogni, Carol M. Devine, and Margaret Jastran. 2006. A Conceptual Model of the Food Choice Process over the Life Course. In *The Psychology of Food Choice*. Frontiers in Nutritional Science Number 3, edited by Richard Shepherd and Monique Raats, pp. 1–18. Centre for Agriculture and Bioscience International, Guildford, United Kingdom.

Sotero, Michelle. 2006. A Conceptual Model of Historical Trauma: Implications for Public Health Practice and Research. *Journal of Health Disparities Research and Practice* 1(1):93–108.

Starr, Arigon. 2012. *Super Indian: Volume One*. Wacky Productions Unlimited, Los Angeles, California.

Steinberg, A. 1989. Holocaust Survivors and Their Children: A Review of the Clinical Literature. In *Healing Their Wounds: Psychotherapy with Holocaust Survivors and Their Families*, edited by Paul Marcus and Alan Rosenberg, pp. 23–48. Praeger Publishers, Westport, Connecticut.

Story, M., M. Evans, R. R. Fabsitz, T. E. Clay, B. Holy Rock, and B. Broussard. 1999. The Epidemic of Obesity in American Indian Communities and the Need for Childhood Obesity-Prevention Programs. *The American Journal of Clinical Nutrition* 69(4 Suppl):747S-754S.

Strakosch, Elizabeth. 2024. "Violence as Care: Indigenous Policy and Settler Colonialism." In *Handbook of Indigenous Public Policy*, edited by Sheryl Lightfoot and Sarah Maddison, pp. 18–34. Edward Elgar Publishing, Cheltenham, United Kingdom. https://www.elgaronline.com/edcollchap/book/9781800377011/book -part-9781800377011-7.xml.

TallBear, Kim. 2013. Genomic Articulations of Indigeneity. *Social Studies of Science* 43(4):509–533. https://doi.org/10.1177/0306312713483893.

Tallbear, Kim. 2019. Being in Relation. In *Messy Eating*, edited by Samantha R. King, Scott Carey, Isabel Macquarrie, Victoria Niva Millious, and Elaine M. Power, pp. 54–67. Fordham University Press, New York. https://doi.org/10.1515/978082 3283675-004.

TallBear, Kim. 2020. Identity Is a Poor Substitute for Relating: Genetic Ancestry, Critical Polyamory, Property, and Relations. In *Routledge Handbook of Critical Indigenous Studies*, edited by Brendan Hokowhitu, Aileen Moreton-Robinson, Linda Tuhiwai-Smith, Chris Andersen, and Steve Larkin, pp. 467–478. Routledge, New York and London. https://www.taylorfrancis.com/chapters/edit/10.4324/978042 9440229-40/identity-poor-substitute-relating-kim-tallbear.

Thomas, Kevin. 2024. The Emergence of a Hypothesized Freedmen Status amongst Black American Reparations Advocates. Available at *Social Science Research Network 4715858*. https://papers.ssrn.com/sol3/papers.cfm?abstract_id=4715858.

Thompson, Ian, Jacqueline Putman, Misty Madbull, Makynna Sharp, Jessica Presley, Alex Jauregui-Dusseau, Kaylee Clyma, and Valarie Blue Bird Jernigan. 2023. The Choctaw Nation's Growing Hope Program. *Health Promotion Practice* 24(6):1080–1082.

Todd, Zoe. 2016. This Is the Life. In *Living on the Land: Indigenous Women's Understanding of Place*, edited by Isabel Altamirano-Jiménez and Nathalie Kermoal, 191–212. Athabasca University Press, Alberta.

Townsend, Marilyn S., Janet Peerson, Bradley Love, Cheryl Achterberg, and Suzanne P. Murphy. 2001. Food Insecurity Is Positively Related to Overweight in Women. *The Journal of Nutrition* 131(6):1738–1745.

Trahant, Mark N. 2018. The Story of Indian Health Is Complicated by History, Shortages & Bouts of Excellence. *Daedalus* 147(2):116–123. https://doi.org/10.1162 /DAED_a_00495.

Trinidad, Alma MO. 2009. Toward Kuleana (Responsibility): A Case Study of a Contextually Grounded Intervention for Native Hawaiian Youth and Young Adults. *Aggression and Violent Behavior* 14(6):488–498.

Tuck, Eve, and K. Wayne Yang. 2012. Decolonization Is Not a Metaphor. *Decolonization: Indigeneity, Education & Society* 1(1):1–40.

Tunbridge, J. E., and G. J. Ashworth. 1996. *Dissonant Heritage: The Management of the Past as a Resource in Conflict*. Wiley-Blackwell, Hoboken, New Jersey. https:// trove.nla.gov.au/version/25914675.

United Nations General Assembly. 2007. *United Nations Declaration on the Rights of Indigenous Peoples: Resolution / adopted by the General Assembly*, A/RES/61/295, October 2, 12:1–18.

United States Bureau of the Census. 2011. American Indian and Alaska Native Heritage Month. Profile America, Facts for Features. Electronic document, https://www.census.gov/newsroom/releases/archives/facts_for_features_special_editions/cb11-ff22.html.

United States Bureau of the Census. 2012. American Community Survey. https://www.census.gov/programs-surveys/acs.

United States Census Bureau. A Look at the Largest American Indian and Alaska Native Tribes and Villages in the Nation, Tribal Areas and States. Electronic document, https://www.census.gov/library/stories/2023/10/2020-census-dhc-a-aian-population.html, accessed August 15, 2024.

United States Census Bureau. Native American Heritage Day: November 24, 2023. Electronic document, https://www.census.gov/newsroom/stories/native-american-heritage-day.html, accessed August 15, 2024.

United States Census Bureau. My Tribal Area. Electronic document, https://www.census.gov/tribal/?aianihh=5590, accessed August 15, 2024.

United States Commission on Civil Rights. 2004. Broken Promises: Evaluating the Native American Health Care System. Electronic document, https://www.usccr.gov/files/pubs/2018/12-20-Broken-Promises.pdf.

United States Department of Agriculture. 2014. Food Distribution Program on Indian Reservations. *Food and Nutrition Service Nutrition Program Fact Sheet.* Electronic document, http://www.fns.usda.gov/sites/default/files/pfs-fdpir.pdf.

United States Department of Agriculture. 2015. USDA to Help 821 Rural Small Businesses Boost Renewable Energy Use, Save on Energy Costs. Press Release 0162.16. National Institute of Food and Agriculture. Electronic document, https://nifa.usda.gov/resource/nifa-strikeforce-map-fy-2010-fy-2016-county-summary.

United States Department of Agriculture. 2023. WIC Breastfeeding Data Local Agency Report. Food and Nutrition Service, The Special Supplemental Nutrition Program for Women, Infants and Children (WIC). Electronic document, https://fns-prod.azureedge.us/wic/breastfeeding-data.

VanDerwarker, Amber M., Jon B. Marcoux, and Kandace D. Hollenbach. 2013. Farming and Foraging at the Crossroads: The Consequences of Cherokee and European Interaction Through the Late Eighteenth Century. *American Antiquity* 78(1):68–88. https://doi.org/10.7183/0002-7316.78.1.68.

Vantrease, Dana. 2013. Commod Bods and Frybread Power: Government Food Aid in American Indian Culture. *Journal of American Folklore* 126(499):55–69.

Ver Ploeg, Michele, and Ilya Rahkovsky. 2016. Recent Evidence on the Effects of Food Store Access on Food Choice and Diet Quality. United States Department of Agriculture, May 2. Electronic document, https://www.ers.usda.gov/amber-waves/2016/may/recent-evidence-on-the-effects-of-food-store-access-on-food-choice-and-diet-quality/.

Vizenor, Gerald. 2008. *Survivance: Narratives of Native Presence.* University of Nebraska Press, Lincoln.

Vizenor, Gerald Robert. 1999. *Manifest Manners: Narratives on Postindian Survivance.* University of Nebraska Press, Lincoln.

Wacquant, Loïc. 2004. Following Pierre Bourdieu into the Field. *Ethnography* 5(4):387–414. https://doi.org/10.1177/1466138104052259.

Wacquant, Loïc J. D., and Pierre Bourdieu. 1992. *An Invitation to Reflexive Sociology.* University of Chicago Press, Illinois. https://www.academia.edu/download/4810 9103/bourdieu2.pdf.

Waldman, Laura. 2023. No Settled Law on Settled Land: Legal Struggles for Native American Land and Sovereignty Rights. *CUNY L. Rev.* 26(2):220–259.

Walls, Melissa L., and Les B. Whitbeck. 2012. The Intergenerational Effects of Relocation Policies on Indigenous Families. *Journal of Family Issues* 33(9): 1272–1293.

Walters, Karina L., Selina A. Mohammed, Teresa Evans-Campbell, Ramona E. Beltrán, David H. Chae, and Bonnie Duran. 2011. Bodies Don't Just Tell Stories, They Tell Histories. *Du Bois Review: Social Science Research on Race* 8(01): 179–189.

Wang, Ning, Xiaodong Zhou, Filemon K. Tan, Morris W. Foster, Frank C. Arnett, and Ranajit Chakraborty. 2004. Genetic Signatures of Pre-Expansion Bottleneck in the Choctaw Population of Oklahoma. *American Journal of Physical Anthropology* 124(4):373–379. https://doi.org/10.1002/ajpa.10363.

Wang, Y. Claire, John Pamplin, Michael W. Long, Zachary J. Ward, Steven L. Gortmaker, and Tatiana Andreyeva. 2015. Severe Obesity in Adults Cost State Medicaid Programs Nearly $8 Billion In 2013. *Health Affairs* 34(11):1923–1931. https://doi.org/10.1377/hlthaff.2015.0633.

Wansink, Brian. 2004. Environmental Factors That Increase the Food Intake and Consumption Volume of Unknowing Consumers. *Annual Review of Nutrition* 24:455–479.

Ward, Zachary J., Sara N. Bleich, Angie L. Cradock, Jessica L. Barrett, Catherine M. Giles, Chasmine Flax, Michael W. Long, and Steven L. Gortmaker. 2019. Projected U.S. State-Level Prevalence of Adult Obesity and Severe Obesity. *New England Journal of Medicine* 381(25):2440–2450. https://doi.org/10.1056/NEJMsa 1909301.

Ward, Zachary J., Sara N. Bleich, Michael W. Long, and Steven L. Gortmaker. 2021. Association of Body Mass Index with Health Care Expenditures in the United States by Age and Sex. *PloS One* 16(3):e0247307. https://doi.org/10.1371/journal .pone.0247307.

Watson, Steve, and Emma Waterton. 2010. Reading the Visual: Representation and Narrative in the Construction of Heritage. *Material Culture Review / Revue de La Culture Matérielle* 71(Spring/Printemps):84–97. https://journals.lib.unb.ca /index.php/MCR/article/view/18377.

Watts, Vanessa. 2013. Indigenous Place-Thought and Agency amongst Humans and Non Humans (First Woman and Sky Woman Go on a European World Tour!). *Decolonization: Indigeneity, Education & Society* 2(1):20–34. https://jps.library .utoronto.ca/index.php/des/article/view/19145.

Wertsch, James. 2011. The Role of Narratives in Commemoration: Remembering as Mediated Action. In *Heritage, Memory and Identity*, edited by Helmut Anheier and Yudhishthir Raj Isar, pp. 25–38. Cultures and Globalization series 4.

Wesley-Esquimaux, Cynthia C., and Magdalena Smolewski. 2004. *Historic Trauma and Aboriginal Healing*. Aboriginal Healing Foundation, Ottowa.

Whitbeck, Les B., Gary W. Adams, Dan R. Hoyt, and Xiaojin Chen. 2004. Conceptualizing and Measuring Historical Trauma among American Indian People. *American Journal of Community Psychology* 33(3/4):119–130.

Wiedman, Dennis. 2012. Native American Embodiment of the Chronicities of Modernity: Reservation Food, Diabetes, and the Metabolic Syndrome among the Kiowa, Comanche, and Apache. *Medical Anthropology Quarterly* 26(4):595–612.

Wiley, Andrea S. 1992. Adaptation and the Biocultural Paradigm in Medical Anthropology: A Critical Review. *Medical Anthropology Quarterly* 6(3):216–236.

Wilkins, David E., and Heidi Kiiwetinepinesiik Stark. 2017. *American Indian Politics and the American Political System*. Rowman & Littlefield, Lanham, Maryland.

Williams, David R., Harold W. Neighbors, and James S. Jackson. 2003. Racial/Ethnic Discrimination and Health: Findings from Community Studies. *American Journal of Public Health* 93(2):200–208.

Williamson, D. A., L. G. Womble, N. L. Zucker, D. L. Reas, M. A. White, D. C. Blouin, and F. Greenway. 2000. Body Image Assessment for Obesity (BIA-O): Development of a New Procedure. *International Journal of Obesity and Related Metabolic Disorders: Journal of the International Association for the Study of Obesity* 24(10):1326–1332.

Williamson, Donald A., C. J. Davis, Sandra M. Bennett, Anthony J. Goreczny, and David H. Gleaves. 1989. Development of a Simple Procedure for Assessing Body Image Disturbances. *Behavioral Assessment* 11(4):433–446.

Willows, Noreen D., Anthony J. G. Hanley, and Treena Delormier. 2012. A Socioecological Framework to Understand Weight-Related Issues in Aboriginal Children in Canada. *Applied Physiology, Nutrition, and Metabolism* 37(1):1–13. https://doi .org/10.1139/h11-128.

Winson, Anthony. 2004. Bringing Political Economy into the Debate on the Obesity Epidemic. *Agriculture and Human Values* 21(4):299–312. https://doi.org/10.1007 /s10460-003-1206-6.

Wolfe, Patrick. 2006. Settler Colonialism and the Elimination of the Native. *Journal of Genocide Research* 8(4):387–409. https://doi.org/10.1080/14623520601056240.

Wood, Peter H. 2006. The Changing Population of the Colonial South: An Overview by Race and Region, 1685–1790. In *Powhatan's Mantle: Indians in the Colonial Southeast*, revised and expanded edition., edited by Gregory A. Waselkov, Peter H. Wood, and Tom Hatley, pp. 57–132. University of Nebraska Press, Lincoln.

Yamada, Seiji, and Wesley Palmer. 2007. An Ecosocial Approach to the Epidemic of Cholera in the Marshall Islands. *Social Medicine* 2(2):79–88.

Yan, Jing, Lin Liu, Guowei Huang, and Peizhong Peter Wang. 2014. The Association between Breastfeeding and Childhood Obesity: A Meta-Analysis. *BMC Public Health* 14(1267). https://doi.org/10.1186/1471-2458-14-1267.

Young, Molly. 2021. Oklahoma Gov. Stitt Won't Renew Hunting, Fishing Compacts with Cherokee, Choctaw Tribes. *The Oklahoman 13 December.* Oklahoma City. https://eu.oklahoman.com/story/news/2021/12/13/oklahoma-tribes-gov-kevin -stitt-cancel-hunting-fishing-compacts-cherokee-choctaw/6496127001/.

Zembylas, Michalinos, and Z. Bekerman. 2008. Education and the Dangerous Memories of Historical Trauma: Narratives of Pain, Narratives of Hope. *Curriculum Inquiry* 38(2):125–154.

INDEX

NOTE: Italicized numbers indicate pages with images or tables.

ABOUT THE AUTHOR

Kasey Jernigan is a Choctaw scholar, anthropologist, and Native American Indigenous studies researcher. She is an assistant professor of American studies and anthropology at the University of Virginia and co-director of the Black and Indigenous Feminist Futures Institute there. She holds a doctorate in medical anthropology and a graduate certificate in Native American Indigenous studies from the University of Massachusetts Amherst, and a master's in public health from the University of Oklahoma Health Sciences Center.